A Framework for Managing POTS

How I took charge of my wellness

& turned my life around

Ysmay Walsh

NFE Books
Austin, Texas

Disclaimer:

This book is not a substitute for medical or nutritional advice. The content provided herein is for educational purposes only. This book is not a substitute for professional medical care. Always seek the advice of your physician or other qualified health care provider with any questions you may have regarding a medical condition or treatment, before undertaking a new health care regimen, and/or before making any lifestyle changes. Never disregard professional medical advice or delay seeking it because of something you have read in this book.

Contents

In memory of Christina

Preface

This book is not for everyone. But it might be for you.

If you are

- living with Postural Orthostatic Tachycardia Syndrome
- sick and tired of being sick and tired
- feeling hopeless
- willing to take control of your situation
- willing to believe there is potentially something you can do
- not willing to be a victim of your illness

Then read on!

Introduction

There are moments in life when suddenly everything changes. One moment you are going about your business and the next moment the foundation of your world is rocked.

You are shaken to your core.

Over time you start to get your sense of balance back; you start to move forward, but you are never the same again.

I was shaken to my core in March 2015 thanks to a beautiful, intelligent, vibrant young woman in Tampa, Florida named Christina Tournant.

After graduating from Osceola Fundamental High School as valedictorian, Christina was accepted to the Massachusetts Institute of Technology. To those who would meet her in passing, it looked like she would lead a charmed life. She was beautiful, smart, and had a bright future ahead of her.

However, Christina had Postural Orthostatic Tachycardia Syndrome (POTS), a relatively uncommon nervous system disorder, which severely restricted her life.

Christina's health took a bad turn in December 2014, but she pushed on. In February she went home from MIT on medical leave. But it soon became too much.

Thursday, March 5, Christina stood atop a parking garage at the Tampa International Airport and sent her Mom a text message: "I love you Mom."

At 8:25pm Christina's body was found where she died after jumping off the top of the parking garage. Christina left a suicide note on the back of a photograph of her with her mother which expressed her regret at not being able to solve the puzzle of her health---the puzzle of POTS.

Christina's death touched me more profoundly than I expected. Reading her story brought me to tears because I've been there. I get it. I have stood on the edge of my own metaphorical parking garage, staring into the abyss.

I understand why Christina jumped.

When I was her age, I thought things would never get better. I thought I would spend my life disabled, unable to walk up stairs, unable to go for a walk in the mall with friends. Some days I could barely get out of bed.

Suicide crossed my mind several times.

I have had POTS since I was a little kid, although I was not diagnosed until I was a teenager. My POTS manifested as a heart problem and when I was a child POTS wasn't really a recognized condition.

After several years – years which included unsuccessful heart surgery and more medications than I can remember - I was finally diagnosed with dysautonomia. (My exact diagnosis is Postural Orthostatic Tachycardia Syndrome and Inappropriate Sinus Tachycardia caused by dysautonomia.)

Deeply depressed as a teenager, rebellious and vulnerable, I wanted to live my life on the edge. I never knew how long I had, or whether or not I would be able to get out of bed the next day.

I wanted to do what I wanted, when I wanted, consequences be damned.

I experimented with drugs, alcohol and smoking, among other reckless behaviors. Anything for a distraction. Anything for a few moments of solace; a few moments where I was not in pain.

Like Christina, I, too, was overwhelmed by POTS. I didn't see how it could get better.

In my early 20s I accepted that I was just going to be sick and tired the rest of my life. At least it was a life. And this acknowledgment, this understanding, suited me for some time.

Eventually I got sick and tired of being sick and tired, and I decided to take matters into my own hands, and I am very glad I did.

I have been fortunate enough to develop a framework that works for me, but it took a lot of work. It has taken me *years* to get to where I am.

This book has been a work in progress since Autumn 2014. It started out as just a chronicle of what I did that worked for me. Eventually, maybe, somewhere down the line I'd publish it. I wasn't really attached to getting it out there.

But then Christina passed and it occurred to me there are so many people suffering that I would be doing a disservice to work on it only as a hobby.

This book explains my framework; the framework that has worked *for me*. What you will read in these pages is what has helped me transform my wellness, and live a life (relatively) free of restrictions.

This book is designed to be a resource for those who are tired of the struggle, tired of being told we just have anxiety, tired of doctors who know less than we do, and sick and tired of being sick and tired! All that being said, *this may not work for you at all*. POTS is a very subjective condition; *we are all different*. We all have different symptoms, challenges, and struggles.

I am not a doctor. I am just a very stubborn patient who figured out how to manage my own wellness. <u>This book is not a substitute for medical advice, and is for educational purposes only. Discuss any lifestyle design changes you wish to make with your trusted medical professionals.</u>

If all you take away from this is that you do not have to be a victim of this horrible condition that crushes people's hopes and dreams, I have done my job.

My Story

I was eight years old when I first had chest pain. It was my brother's and grandmother's birthday – they were both born on July 16 – and we were all sitting around the table having cake. I clutched my chest and started crying. My parents whisked me off to the hospital where - much to everybody's dismay - we didn't get very many answers.

After many tests, Children's Hospital visits and doctor's appointments, I was officially diagnosed with supraventricular tachycardia. Supraventricular tachycardia (or SVT as it's most commonly known) is an abnormal heart rhythm that starts in the upper chambers of the heart. SVT can cause chest pain, shortness of breath, fainting, fatigue, and palpitations.

For years that was my official diagnosis and I had to adjust my life accordingly. I couldn't go to gym class. I couldn't run. I had trouble walking up stairs. I couldn't lift or carry things. I felt like an invalid, but that's a feeling you quickly get used to when you don't have a choice.

When I was 18 my health suddenly went from bad to worse. I ended up hospitalized for SVT and atrial fibrillation. The solution? Surgery. An exploratory procedure called an electrophysiology study accompanied by radio frequency catheter ablation.

The doctors used medication to keep me awake during the procedure. They were trying to recreate my SVTs and a-fib; I needed to be awake so I could tell them when I was in pain.

I remember lying on a surgical bed staring up at a lovely mural of hot air balloons that some talented artist painted on the ceiling. I remember thinking about how nice it would be to just float away, and this would all be over with.

And then something weird happened; the electrophysiologist said a phrase you never want to hear during a procedure like that: "Hm...that's interesting."

Just like that the procedure was finished, and I was whisked off to recovery, where I don't really remember much of anything thanks to a fabulous drug called Versed. When I followed up with my cardiologist the following week I finally learned what the "Hm..." was all about.

Turns out, my heart is fine. Not only is my heart fine, it's the picture of cardiac health.

This brought up a new question. Why am I having cardiac symptoms if my heart is the picture of health?

Several more months of tests and I was diagnosed with dysautonomia, a dysfunction of the autonomic nervous system. I have been diagnosed with both Postural Orthostatic Tachycardia Syndrome and Inappropriate Sinus Tachycardia in the years since.

The autonomic nervous system is responsible for making sure our involuntary bodily functions continue to function properly. It's responsible for regulating heart rate, blood pressure, respiratory rate, and the gastrointestinal system. When you have dysautonomia, things get a little wacky and they do so at random times.

Dysautonomia International estimates that POTS impacts between 1,000,000 - 3,000,000 Americans, with 80% of patients being women. The severity of POTS varies from patient to patient, as does the number of - and intensity of - symptoms each patient exhibits. Because of how POTS presents in each patient, there is no cure. Treatments focus on treating each symptom as it arises.

Life with dysautonomia is a constant battle being waged between wanting to be healthy, happy, and productive, and not being able to get out of bed. The quality of life for POTS patients has been compared to that of a patient with kidney failure who is on dialysis.

When Christina Tournant committed suicide it was because she couldn't deal with it anymore. That struck a chord with me. If only she knew it can get better. If only she had hope...maybe she would have kept fighting.

I was in her shoes. I've been there. I get it. I understand the desire to end it all...not because I actually wanted to die, but because it would just be easier.

One thing all POTSies have in common is being sick and tired of being sick and tired *all the time*.

It gets especially frustrating when you look at people in your life who are healthy; who are normal. I'm sure you have someone in your life who even abuses their body. They run on very little sleep. They have very little structure. They eat complete crap and abuse substances. They do all this – and more – with zero consequences.

I have some people like this in my life, too. When I watch them stay up late, get drunk, smoke a pack of cigarettes a day, get 4 hours of sleep, work for 12 hours, and still be perfectly fine, I feel sad, envious, and, yes, even a little outraged. I don't feel these things because I want to be able to abuse my body, but because I can't be even a *little* careless without dire consequences.

And you know what? Sometimes it makes me want to scream at them, "You have a fabulous body! It functions the way it's supposed to! And what do you do? You abuse it! I would do *anything* to have a body that functions normally, and here you are actively destroying yours."

As a fellow POTSie you probably understand my outrage.

For a long time I was unable to work; I was barely able to stand. I had to sleep at least 12 hours a day. Over time I got to a point where I was able to work, but working was so hard on my body I had to then sleep for 14 hours a day.

Then one day, I decided I had had enough. It all started because my husband and I moved into our first place together. This apartment was a tiny little third floor walk-up with 47 steps to get to our apartment. It was *a big problem* since stairs suck for POTSies.

After spending yet another 20 minutes sitting at the top of the stairs after walking home one day, I decided, "I am sick and tired of being sick and tired, and I'm going to do something about it." POTS be damned.

I had some limited experience with yoga at this point, and after doing more research I learned yoga helps calm the parasympathetic nervous system. I had heard rumors about it several times over the years, but I never really thought anything of it because I never heard it from a qualified source.

One day I went to Walmart, got myself a cheap yoga mat, and started following Erin Motz's 30 Day Yoga Challenge videos on YouTube.

It took me more like 90 days, but the results were astounding.

I started sleeping like a normal person. My migraines went away. My chest pain become less frequent. I had more energy. I could breathe! I could walk up stairs! I could carry stuff! I felt like a new woman.

Because I WAS a new woman.

About a year after starting yoga, I started to notice that when I ate meat I felt worse and had more cardiac symptoms. So I quit eating meat cold turkey. (Pun intended!)

After adopting this new lifestyle, my life was vastly improved in ways my doctors didn't think was possible.

Because of the radical shift I experienced in my wellness through yoga and holistic practices, I started 42Yogis.com in April 2014 to help others achieve wellness, too.

While yoga is what really changed my life, I never would have tried to experiment with my wellness if it weren't for a man named Tim Ferriss. Because, well, let's be honest: I had given up.

Tim Ferriss is an entrepreneur, investor, author, and body-hacker. I read his book *The 4 Hour Work Week* shortly after it came out, and it transformed the way I look at business. About 5 years ago my then-roommate came home with Ferriss' book *The Four Hour Body*.

I first dismissed it as a book for men who are trying to get jacked, but after perusing the pages I started to understand. It's not about body building. It's about biohacking – experimenting on your body in order to create abundant wellness.

The Four Hour Body was interesting, but for months I didn't do anything with it. I moved to Austin, Texas, suddenly and stopped focusing on things like a sleep schedule and eating right during a major life transition.

Once I got out of my routines, my health took a serious downturn.

Then, after moving from Texas to New York - I relocated across the country three times that year - I started having major problems with my sleep. Sleep has always been a struggle for me; I was even a sleepwalker as a kid. My sleep has never been normal.

I remembered Ferriss' book had a great chapter about sleep, so I bought another copy as mine had vanished somewhere among the moves. I figured if all I got out of the book was how to sleep better, it would have been money well spent.

While I didn't implement a lot of the strategies regarding weight loss and fat loss, I got so much more than what I paid for. I regained the motivation and inspiration to take my health into my own hands.

I realized you don't have to rely on doctors and Western medicine to make you healthy. You don't have to take 900 pills a day to create wellness. Even if you have POTS and are struggling to get out of bed every day, you have all the tools you need to cultivate more wellness. I'm not saying you'll be running marathons; hell, I'm not running marathons (yet), but we *can* learn how to make the most of the hand we've been dealt.

Getting to where I am has been a struggle. It has taken a lot of work, and a lot of steps backward (followed by very small steps forward) to get to where I am now.

I am now walking up stairs, playing tennis, sleeping like a normal person, and training for a 5K.

Never would I have thought I could be this healthy.

There was a time I was severely depressed, much like Christina. I had no hope; I saw no light at the end of the tunnel. It is because of Christina that I have decided to share my tips, my method, that got my POTS under control.

In the following pages you will find the framework that has worked for me, and I will guide you through potentially *creating your own*.

For POTSies there is no one-size-fits-all solution for our health and wellness. If you have been going to doctors with any degree of regularity, you know the treatments for POTS tend to have radically different results from patient to patient.

Your body is your own body; it is unique, for better or worse. Anybody who tells you all you have to do is implement their step-by-step routine and your POTS will be gone has either been endowed with a gift from the gods... or is simply lying.

While I can't give you a step-by-step implementation plan, I *can* teach you how to develop your own wellness framework so you can start to have fewer POTSie days.

You need a framework that works for you, your lifestyle, and your body. *Developing your own framework is what this is all about.*

This book is not your average health and wellness book. This book is a framework designed to help you have fewer POTSie days. This book explains my story, my framework, and guides you through *creating one of your own*.

I am not a medical professional, nor do I make any claims to be. While working on this book, I reached out to a number of medical and nutritional professionals to get their input, and their explanations about why what I have done has helped me. You will see these professionals quoted in various places in this book.

Any errors or omissions in their statements are mine alone. Remember, this is not intended as medical advice. Speak with your own trusted healthcare professionals and ask them any questions you may have about your individual needs and options.

Three Pillars of Wellness

In my experience, there are three pillars to wellness:

1. Goals
2. Biohacking
3. Lifestyle Design

Once these three pillars are constructed, you can develop your framework. But without these three pillars, your framework will collapse before you even get started.

Goals
Goals are something many of us struggle with. We want to do something, we want to improve somehow, but we aren't entirely sure what it is we are striving for. We are bad about creating specific goals. Specificity is what separates those who achieve their goals from those who don't. The more specific your wellness goals, the more likely you are to achieve them.

Biohacking
Biohacking is the process of experimenting with your habits from an analytical perspective to cultivate better wellness. When I first started biohacking, I didn't know that's what I was doing. I started logging what I ate, when I ate, how I felt, my exercise, my heart rate, my blood pressure, my blood sugar, and using that data to make informed decisions in order to change my wellness. This is biohacking!

Lifestyle Design
It's not enough to have a wellness goal and to biohack your way to it. You need to be able to create a lifestyle that is conducive to the long-term implementation of your new habits. For example, you won't be very successful in implementing a new, healthier, eating routine if you keep buying junk food. You won't be very successful with getting to bed at a regular hour if you don't make adjustments to other parts of your day.

Together we will construct these three pillars and then we will work on developing your framework.

The framework you are going to develop impacts four key areas of your life:

> Sleep
> Food and Drink
> Exercise
> Personal Development

Sleep
Sleep is the key to everything. Without supportive sleep our wellness suffers. When I have poor sleep, I get migraines, chest pain, dizziness, and lethargy so overwhelming I can barely get off the couch.

Food and Drink
Food plays a much larger role in managing my POTS than I expected. I only discovered the importance of managing diet in 2010, however I did not take it seriously until 2013. Most people do not have the symptoms we get from food. If I eat too much gluten, I get palpitations. If I eat too many carbs, I get palpitations. If I eat meat, I get palpitations. But I didn't discover these all at once. I discovered my triggers over time, and you can too.

Exercise
Exercise is so very important, but so very hard to come by. Us POSTsies have to be flexible enough to manage our time, but take a break and reschedule based on our health. If we exercise, we risk a flare that can last days. I have been fortunate to find exercise that I can do without getting a flare.

Personal Development
We may have a really crappy health condition, but that doesn't make us less of a person. That doesn't mean we are less than our friends or family. We are complete human beings with goals, desires, dreams, and a vibrant soul. Ignoring your personal development because of POTS is one of the worst things you can do. Ignoring your passions and stifling your soul will lead to depression, which can trigger POTS flares.

This book is designed to give you a framework for transforming your health and wellness, but it isn't one-size-fits-all. I can only guide you. *You have to implement it in a way that helps you and transforms your life and wellness, and only you and your medical team will be able to know what that is.*

But before we get started...

This is not going to be the most well-received chapter of this book, and I understand I am bound to make some enemies among readers before they even get into the valuable content I have to share. But, this is necessary:

Don't be a victim.

You may not have a victim mentality but many people I've met with POTS do, and it is their biggest roadblock. It is what is standing in their way of making the most of their situation and living a better life.

I have been in several support groups over the years, and something I keep seeing time and time again is patients acting like victims.[*] People acting as if since POTS has happened to them, it's nothing they can control, or change, or handle.

"Life sucks. Woe is me." It's an easy mental pattern to fall into. You stop being able to do things you could do before. You struggle to get up in the morning. You struggle to keep your heart rate down. You struggle to walk up the stairs. Medications don't always work. Doctors don't always have answers.

It's easy to feel like this just happened to you and you therefore have no hope of living a normal life. It's easy to be overwhelmed by the struggle, the pain, the discomfort, the ache in your soul that comes with having to disappoint your family once again.

It is easy to feel disempowered.

But if you are feeling disempowered, I want you to remember that you are not the only one! We all feel disempowered. Everybody who has a chronic illness has had a time when they felt disempowered. I've been there!

---

[*] For what it's worth, I asked some friends of mine who are in cancer and other support groups, and it appears the victim mentality is not specific to dysautonomia patients.

However, it is important to recognize your health and wellness will never improve until you accept that the victim mentality does not serve you in the long run.

There are several short-term "benefits" of having a victim mentality, including:

Attention
You can almost always get sympathy and attention from others when you are living and acting as a victim.

Living in your comfort zone
You don't have to take any unnecessary risks – emotional or physical. You can use your health as the perfect excuse not to do something that you don't want to do.

Not taking responsibility
Taking responsibility for the struggles in your life is not fun. Let's be honest: adulting sucks. When you live with a victim mentality you get to blame everything that sucks in your life on your health, even if your health is not actually to blame.

The problem with being a victim is that you lose your power.

When you adopt the mindset of, "This horrible thing happened to me and I can't do anything about it," you are surrendering. You are admitting defeat. You surrender your power and your strength to this condition.

When you admit defeat you stop fighting. You stop trying to improve, change, grow, and adapt. And then what happens? You endlessly suffer, and struggle, and live in a state of despair.

That doesn't benefit you. That doesn't help you to become a better person...a healthier person.

If you really want to be healthier...

If you really want to be able to get some of the benefits I talked about…

If you really want to transform your life…

You have to get rid of the victim mentality.

You have to sacrifice the short-term "benefits" of being a victim for the greater good: your long-term health.

If you are not willing to stop being a victim, then put this book down, and stop wasting your time. Because here's the thing: If you are not willing to cowgirl up, take responsibility for your life, take responsibility for your actions and your choices, and choose to live an empowered life *despite* the health struggles you are enduring on a daily basis, I cannot help you.

Nobody can help you until you stop standing in your own way.

So how do you do that? How do you stop being a victim?

You start by forgiving yourself. You are not to blame for what happened to you. You are not to blame for POTS. POTS is not a punishment for something you did. POTS is not bad karma. Stop blaming yourself and stop seeing yourself as an inferior human being. Forgive yourself for the heartache you've caused yourself, and the hurtful thoughts you may have about your body.

You start by accepting some responsibility for your life and your actions. Yes, POTS is miserable. But does your life have to be as bad as it is? Do you have to let POTS drain you of that which makes you, *you*? Do you have to let it dull your sparkle? No.

You start by giving thanks for what you do have. There are so many people in the world less fortunate than you, and you are truly, truly blessed. It does not feel like it sometimes; it may not even feel like it now, but you are truly blessed. Give thanks. Be grateful. Display gratitude. Say a prayer of thanks in the morning, which will set a positive tone for your day and start to undo some of the negative thoughts you have. You can do this even if you are not in any way religious. Just hold a yourself in a moment of gratitude to start the day.

And then start to see the blessings in the situation. You have had to learn, and grow, and expand your mind, and learn about the world of medicine, and deepen your connection to your body in ways that most people never will. You have met people in support groups you wouldn't have met otherwise. You have had experiences that lift you up and enhance your spirit that you would not have otherwise.

If you're still not willing to stop being a victim, stop reading right now, because you're just going to waste your energy.

HOWEVER, if you're willing to stop being a victim, and you're willing to become empowered and take charge, go on to the next chapter for the three rules you must abide by if you're going to make this work.

The Rules

There are three rules that you should abide by when trying to take charge of your health and wellness.

1. Listen to your body.

Everybody is different and every *body* is different. This is especially true of POTSies. While we all have similar symptoms, we all have circumstances that make the condition uniquely ours. For better or worse, we all have a different experience of this condition.

Just because something worked for me does not necessarily mean it will work for you. You may have trouble with some things that worked easily for me, and some things that took more effort for me may come easily to you. Listen to your body above all else.

2. Talk to your doctor.

Before you undertake any change in your health and wellness, discuss it with your doctor. Whether that change is something you've read here, or learned elsewhere, discuss it with your trusted medical professionals *first*.

I am not a medical professional, and I did not discuss all the changes I made with my doctors due to the simple fact that for years I did not have health insurance, and could not afford to go to a doctor. Talk to your doctors!

3. Be patient with yourself.

Many people can make a new habit or break an old one in 21 days. Dr. Maxwell Maltz was the first to discover this. Dr. Maxwell Maltz, a plastic surgeon, noticed it took his patients 21 days to cease feeling phantom sensations from amputated limbs. His curiosity was piqued, and after more research he discovered it takes 21 days to build a new habit, suggesting it takes that long for the new pathways to be built in the brain.

It takes me 42 days to break a bad habit and make a new one. That is six weeks. 21 days is too few for me. It's too easy for me to have a misstep on day 25 and get out of my healthy habit.

As a POTSie, it may take you longer simply because you don't have the same level of energy from one day to the next. You may find it takes you anywhere from 21 days to 42 days – or even longer! – to make new habits and change your health. It can seem overwhelming, and this overwhelm can be quite depressing. Be patient with yourself, and let yourself grow and change in your own time.

Getting Started

Before your health can grow and evolve, you need to put in some legwork, and spend some time working on these three areas:

Goals
Biohacking
Lifestyle Design

Setting a goal is important to keep you on track, move forward, and motivate yourself towards success.

In order to achieve your goals, you need to spend some time on biohacking to make some changes and find that which does not serve you.

Once you have the data from biohacking, you need to focus on lifestyle design to make sure you can implement the changes you discovered are necessary in achieving your goal.

Goals

Goals are a powerful tool for achieving anything. You have probably set goals in your life, but have you set any goals for your wellness?

Perhaps you have, but without making essential changes to your lifestyle, you probably weren't successful in achieving them. Setting wellness goals is essential if you want to kick POTS to the curb.

Studies show those who write down their goals are far more likely to achieve them. But most people never learn how to create goals. That's what we're going to work on now.

I want you to get a piece of paper and a pen, and for the next 60 seconds, make a list of all the goals that come to mind. No matter what they are.

Some examples:

- Walk with the dog
- Hold forearm plank for 2 minutes
- Get up early in the morning
- Have lots of energy
- Get on a more regular sleep schedule
- Go to work without getting a migraine
- Not have to take a nap every day
- Sleep through the night
- Wake up feeling rested
- Carry a laundry basket up the stairs
- Have enough energy to run around after the kids
- Be able to eat without digestive issues
- Be more productive at work
- Reduce palpitations

Whatever it is. Write down all your wellness goals that come to mind.

You might have 10 things on the list that would be nice for you to achieve. Or maybe you only have one. If you have more than five spend the next 30 seconds crossing out every goal that doesn't completely resonate with you.

Now cross out every goal that's on your list that you want to achieve for the sake of pleasing somebody else.

For example, do you want to be more productive at work for you or because your boss is a jerk who makes you feel guilty? All too often we write down things we think we want to achieve, but we only want to achieve it to make someone else happy. When we try to do something for someone else, we are generally less likely to be successful.

And let's be honest here: we deserve to do things for ourselves, not for others.

Spend just 30 seconds crossing out the goals that are for other people. Timing is key here. Listen to your intuition and make snap decisions.

Look at the goals you have left.

Most goal setting experts will tell you to rearrange the goals in order of priority. What do you *really* want to achieve? That works great if you are making business goals or productivity goals. But wellness is a little bit different.

When you're making wellness goals consider this:

What goal – if achieved – will make all the other goals easier?

What item will make the rest fall into place? What item will be essential in ensuring long-term success with the other goals?

Let's suppose your goal list looks like this:

- Get up early in the morning
- Have lots of energy

- Be able to go for a walk with the dog
- Wake up feeling rested
- Get on a more regular sleep schedule

Getting up early sounds great, but is this list really doable at this juncture?

If you're a night owl – as so many POTSies seem to be – getting up early is going to be a big struggle. You won't wake up feeling rested, and during the day you won't have very much energy. Ask yourself WHY you want to get up early.

In this example, your number one goal should be to get on a more regular sleep schedule. That one goal – if achieved – will make it easier for you to accomplish the others. If you're on a more regular sleep schedule, it will be easier for you to wake up feeling rested. It will be easier for you to get up early.

While getting on a more regular sleep schedule might not seem like it will do much for dog walking, it will make the other goals on the list more doable. And, if you have more energy, you might be more inclined to take the dog for a walk.

When I first did this exercise, my list looked something like this:

- Get up early in the morning
- Get on a more regular sleep schedule
- Go for a jog
- Eat more regularly
- Have more energy

By rearranging my list so having a more regular sleep schedule was my number one goal, the others became much easier. It was easier for me to get up early in the morning. It was easier for me to have a meal schedule. My energy levels went up, and it became more likely I would workout.

As you are polishing your goals, make sure they are specific. Specificity is what separates those who achieve their goals from those who don't. The more specific your wellness goals, the more likely you are to achieve them.

Don't say, "Get up early in the morning." That's not specific enough. That was one of my mistakes early on. Instead say, "Get up at 7am and be ready to start my work day by 9am."

Make sure you have a realistic date to accomplish the goal. Goals that do not have a date associated with them are too nebulous. It's too easy to wander off course. A date will hold you accountable. It's important to note once again that things often take longer for POTSies.

Take that into account when you are setting your date. It is unrealistic to expect to be able to turn your life around overnight. That will only lead to discouragement.

"At the end of 6 weeks I will get up at 7am and be ready to start my work day by 9am."

That is a realistic goal. That is something that could be achieved.

To ensure goal success, it might help to share your goal with someone. But proceed with caution. In 2010, entrepreneur Derek Sivers famously said telling someone your goals makes you less likely to achieve them because psychologically the act of talking about the goal feels almost as rewarding as accomplishing the goal.

However, only you know if this is the case for you. Only you know if you are more likely to achieve it if you have someone cheering you on. If you do share your goal, I recommend you do so with people who understand what you're going through and have a vested interested in helping you achieve your goal.

Biohacking

Biohacking is the process of experimenting with your habits from an analytical perspective to cultivate better wellness.

When I first started biohacking, I didn't know that's what I was doing. I started logging what I ate, when I ate, how I felt, my exercise, my heart rate, my blood pressure, my blood sugar, and using that data to make informed decisions in order to change my wellness. This is biohacking!

Biohacking all starts with data collection. If something can be tracked it can be changed. But it is unrealistic to expect to be able to make any reasonable, sustainable change without data. You need to know where you are in order to get where you are going. Trying to make long-term changes without data is like trying to run a marathon without knowing where the starting line is.

I recommend a week of data collection for most goals before you try to start making substantial changes. Yes, yes, you may be feeling like, "C'mon! I want to start now!" But believe me when I tell you that you will be much more successful in achieving these goals when you put in the work and collect the data.

There so many wellness programs out there that ask you to jump right in without taking any time to evaluate where you are. As I said, that sounds like trying to run a marathon without knowing where the starting line is!

You can't get rid of food that doesn't serve you until you get the data about what foods those are. If you want to get on an earlier sleep schedule, you probably only have a vague idea at exactly what time you go to bed and exactly what time you get up unless you've already been tracking this.

For the next week start tracking everything. As a POTSie I have discovered everything can affect our wellness, even things we didn't think about, so I suggest you track *everything*.

You may have a general idea of your daily habits and meals, but there is power in seeing it in black and white. Writing it down gets these vague concepts you have about your wellness and eating habits out of your head. When you can see it, you're more likely to hold yourself accountable, and I venture you might even have a moment where you say, "Oh, I didn't know I do that."

At minimum, track sleep, beverages, food, meds, heart rate, energy levels, mood, outdoor temperature, and relative humidity. It is important to track not only what you do, but the conditions under which you do it, and how each item makes you feel.

You can write this down on a piece of paper, in a notebook, or keep all the information in a spreadsheet. However you manage the data, make sure it is somewhere you can access it easily.

Much of the tracking can be made a bit easier thanks to the use of technology.

I invested in a FitBit Charge HR. It tracks my sleep and my heart rate automatically. I discovered I didn't get nearly as much sleep as I need and my heart rate was all over the place. The FitBit dashboard has some awesome charts that let you see what's going on, and you can export the data to spreadsheets for your doctors or for your own personal use.

Other wellness trackers work in a similar manner.

The rest of it is a little bit more tedious. But it is essential. What makes it easier for me is to jot everything down in a tiny notebook or on a piece of paper on the desk, and then transfer to a spreadsheet with my sleep and heart rate data.

It's especially important to track your food. It surprised me to discover that what I eat has a major impact on my health and wellness. I can trigger or avoid POTS flares by adjusting my diet.

Keep track not only of what you eat, but how it makes you feel afterward.

For example, if you drink a can of ginger ale, it might help your nausea, but it might make you feel sluggish. If you have cereal for breakfast, it might briefly satisfy hunger, but you might feel hungry and tired a few hours later.

Track the following things:

1. Date/time of eating (or drinking anything other than water)
2. Item you ate or drank
3. Serving size (totally OK to guesstimate at this point)
4. How you felt while you were eating
5. How you felt immediately afterwards
6. How you felt 30 minutes, 60 minutes, and 90 minutes later
7. Any POTS symptoms after eating, no matter how tiny.

This is not your average food log. We're not tracking carbs, fat, or calories right now. We are purely tracking what you're eating and how it makes you feel. And that is it. Over time you will begin to notice what foods are triggers and what foods aren't.

I came to this realization about six years ago when I was out to dinner. I ordered the potato leek soup, and about 10 minutes after eating I had a flare. My date said, "Have you ever noticed you have an episode after you eat carbs?"

And – embarrassingly – no, I hadn't noticed! I was just eating the food that sounded good; not the food that was good for me.

Before you start making any changes to your diet, I strongly encourage you to put in the effort and spend time tracking your food. Figure out what works for you. Making changes without having any data about where you currently are is like trying to run a marathon without knowing where the starting line is.

After you have been logging your food for a while, you'll begin to see patterns. You will be able to see what foods don't make you feel well afterward.

Again, I don't ask you to count calories. Caloric intake is not my concern, and it shouldn't necessarily be your concern either. Your primary concern should be, "Does this food make me feel well or unwell?"

While I do use MyFitnessPal, I do not use it to keep track of calories. I use MyFitnessPal as an easy way to log everything I eat when I'm on the go. I can transfer it to a spreadsheet later.

I focus on eating food that my body likes. I don't just eat something because I'm craving it. I am mindful of the way I will feel after I eat, instead of just how I will feel while I am eating.

With POTS, we have to be very careful to only eat things that are supportive of our well-being, not destructive to it. It is important that it doesn't cause POTS symptoms.

For example, I don't like the way I feel after drinking coffee, soda, or alcohol, so I don't drink those things.

I don't like the way I feel after having a carb-heavy meal, so I don't eat a lot of carbs in one sitting.

I don't like the way I feel after eating too much gluten, so I don't eat too much gluten in one sitting.

I don't like the way I feel after eating meat, so I don't eat meat.

Getting rid of each of these items has improved my POTS.

To find what works for you, collect your data for about a week. Don't make any substantial changes right now. Just gather data. I know this can be frustrating because you want to start feeling healthier *now*. Believe me, I get it. But without structure, your attempts to manage your POTS symptoms are going to be difficult at best and a failure at worst.

After a week of tracking, move into experimentation. With your goal in mind, write down three experiments you can conduct on yourself in the coming week.

Your experiments could be:

- Replacing coffee with Bulletproof Tea
- Eating more roughage instead of fruit
- Lowering your gluten
- Eating less meat

If you want to get better sleep with less morning fatigue, your experiments could include:

- Restorative yoga before bed
- Shower before bed or after waking
- Having protein before bed and after waking
- Progressive relaxation

Whatever the experiments are, make sure they are trackable. As with any good experiment, you must track the data or you won't know if these things work.

I personally recommend experimenting with every aspect of your life. We are creatures of habit, so we will keep doing something long after the habit has stopped serving us.

I have experimented with the following to find what works for me:

- Gluten
- Carbs
- Protein
- Salt
- Electrolytes
- Binaural beats

- Meditation
- Spinning
- Several styles of yoga
- What kind of tea I drink at different times of the day

Once you start tracking your habits and experimenting with different habits, you'll start to get a comprehensive picture of what works for you and what doesn't work for you.

It bears repeating: as you experiment, you *must* keep tracking the data. This is crucial. If you replaced your afternoon orange with a bowl of kale, how did you feel afterward? What was your energy level like? What was your mood like?

Remember: if something is tracked it can be changed.

Lifestyle Design

This is where it gets fun. You have your goals and you have at least a week's worth of data, and you have done your week of experimentation.

Now, we're going to start working on your lifestyle design.

Language

Before you can expect to achieve your wellness goals, before you can expect to make substantial changes to your lifestyle design, you need to change your language.

I believe that changing your language can change your life. How you think about yourself, how you speak about yourself, how you speak to others (including your tone and attitude!) can influence your actions and worldview in ways you don't even realize.

Here are two examples.

Because I have had dysautonomia my whole life (well, since I was a little kid, but it feels like my whole life!), I used to think, "I can't do that," or "I just want to be normal." I used those two thoughts to keep myself from doing things like yoga or walking. That thinking is toxic. I was telling myself that I am less than everybody else, which is simply untrue.

I may have some health problems, but I have all my fingers, arms, legs, and toes. There is absolutely no reason why I can't cultivate wellness for myself. And when I realized this, I started to do just that. I got a cheap yoga mat at Walmart, I found some yoga videos on YouTube, and I started doing yoga in my living room. It literally changed my life. But it wouldn't have happened if I kept telling myself, "I am less."

Here's my second example. Last year I had a meeting with a business consultant. We were talking about things that I have been struggling with in my business, and she pointed out that I kept saying, "It's hard in this industry." I had been limiting myself by thinking about purely what is common practice in the yoga industry, and that was limiting my success.

When I cut the phrase "It's hard in this industry" from my thoughts and speech, I started to look at my business differently. As a result, I have started to implement business practices and skills I learned from my experience in other industries.

Starting today I want you to take a hard look at the language you use to refer to yourself, whether aloud or not.

I want you to look at the language you use when you speak about your job, about your personal relationships, your health, your intelligence, your abilities, your body, and your POTS. You are *not* less than everybody else. You are *not* inferior. You are *not* a victim.

Do not continue to tell yourself that you are.

I suggest you get a small notebook that will fit in your pocket and use that to track your language throughout the day, or use a note-taking app on your phone. At the end of the day, review your language, and make a note of the general tone in your notebook.

Making Long Term Changes to Your Lifestyle Design

Today is the start of a new you.

Think about this mantra:

> *Today I will let go of my past regrets and allow myself to embrace positive change. I will trust in the process of healing and growth, and move forward into my radiant future.*

The implementation process includes making changes to all areas of your life. This can be scary and intimidating, and you may read the following chapters and feel as if there is no way you are ever going to be able to do this. But I ask you to refer back to Rule #3: be patient with yourself.

Food

According to a 2012 report (Howraa Abed, 2012), "Changing diet and eating habits and increasing fluid intake help people with POTS. Eating small meals has been said to reduce the severity of postprandial hypotension, because the amount of blood required for digestion is reduced."

When we eat, blood is directed to the digestive system. The more we eat, the more blood is required for digestion. By reducing the size of our meals, the amount of blood required for digestion is reduced. This can help us from feeling lethargic and dizzy after a meal.

Also important to consider is the type of food we eat. Not all food is created equal, and not all food affects our body the same way. Complex carbohydrates affect our body differently than simple carbohydrates.

"When you spike your blood sugar, usually from eating simple carbohydrates or sugars without fiber to slow down digestion, you send a confusing hormonal message through your system that is very similar to stress," says Dr. Mark Menolascino.

Dr. Menolascino is an internist with over 25 years of experience, having completed his Internal Medicine Specialist Training at the Mayo Clinic in Arizona after graduating medical school.

The types of food we eat are important in balancing our hormones. Whenever our hormones are out of balance, POTS symptoms can flare. A mistake many people make when it comes to their diet is underestimating the importance of their hormones, especially insulin.

"Insulin has been shown to increase sympathetic activity and the resting heart rate of individuals in small studies," explains Dr. Bernard Ashby, an attending cardiologist and assistant professor of medicine at Columbia University's Division of Cardiology at Mount Sinai Medical Center.

"Insulin promotes the absorption of glucose, a form of carbohydrate, from the blood and therefore is increased with the ingestion of carbohydrates," Dr. Ashby continues. "This is why adhering to a low carbohydrate diet can decrease insulin levels in the blood stream which in turn decreases the sympathetic activity and heart rate."

"A thoughtful nutrition plan prevents the high glycemic index and load from altering cortisol and causing insulin surges," agrees Dr. Menolascino. "Feed your body on nutrition that balances your adrenals and thyroid, and your energy levels will often follow."

Cortisol can be detrimental for POTSies. When cortisol is released it triggers the autonomic nervous system; it can exacerbate POTS symptoms by raising the heart rate and blood pressure, and constricting the small airways (bronchioles) in the lungs. (Understanding the Stress Response, 2011)

Did you see these responses to items in your food log?

Meal Planning

Many people are hesitant to cook or do any meal planning, but when you're trying to get serious about your wellness, you have to be serious about what you eat. That starts with cooking.

"I think people are intimidated by the kitchen," says Liza Baker, Certified Integrative Nutrition Health Coach. "They didn't learn to cook, and after watching the cooking shows, they get even more scared, 'I could never do that!'

"As much as I love them," Baker continues, "I think that cooking shows have done us a great disservice. Michael Pollan writes in *Cooked* that the average American spends 27 minutes making dinner, less time than it takes to watch an episode of *Iron Chef*."

"Another big barrier is a lack of time management/organization skills: our fast-paced, tech-driven lifestyle has made us all somewhat ADD," Baker adds.

If you're strapped for time (and honestly, who isn't?), meal planning can be the answer. Meal planning sounds tedious, and it certainly can be the first couple times you do it, but once you get into the habit, it is very useful to POTSies.

The benefits of meal planning include:

- Making sure you're eating food that is supportive to your health.
- Sticking to a budget when at the grocery store.
- Never wondering what's for dinner.

"Having a properly stocked kitchen is the single most important thing you can do to get nutritious meals on the table with minimal effort," says Michelle Dudash, registered dietitian and nutritionist, Cordon Bleu-certified chef and columnist of DishwithDudash.com.

"That doesn't mean you have to have *a lot* of food, just the *right* foods," Dudash continues.

"For example, keep one type of whole-grain rice on hand at all times, a couple types of legumes, like chickpeas, and always have at least one type of dinnertime vegetable," advises Dudash. "Then, no matter if you planned out actual meals, you always have the essential ingredients needed to throw together a nourishing, balanced meal."

Baker agrees, "One skill I like to teach my clients is that of starting from a well-stocked pantry and understanding what they can create from it - it's rather the reverse of what most of us do, which is start from a recipe, think, 'Oh, I have to run to the store for x, y, z,' then come home and follow the recipe to the letter.

"We are very recipe-bound," adds Baker, "and that costs us a lot of time and money in the long run, making cooking feel unappealing and inefficient."

Another challenge many people have is dealing with picky eaters. As a POTSie, you probably don't have a lot of time and energy as it is, and the last thing you want to do is cook four different meals for four different people. That can make cooking and meal planning seem insurmountable.

"I think it's a trap parents fall into, feeling as though they need to cook three to four different meals - that, too, makes cooking from scratch at home seem difficult," says Baker. "My solution has been to always make enough that any one of us can make a meal out of the offerings.

"For example, I don't eat carbs for dinner, but my husband and son do, so I always have an option for them; my daughter might not like the vegetable offered, but there are carb and protein options that can make up a full meal; my son might not like the protein offered, but he can make a meal of carbs and vegetables," Baker explains.

"We do a lot of 'buffet' meals: soupy noodles, baked potatoes, pastas, tacos with all the fixings that people can choose to eat (or not)," continues Baker. "Don't like anything on offer? There are leftovers in the fridge you can heat."

I think that's one of the most important things to remember. You don't have a lot of energy anyway. POTS takes a toll, and, guess what? You're not a personal chef. You should be cooking the foods that are supportive for you, and it may sound harsh, but try not to worry overly much about what the people in your life will or will not eat.

Of course, there are some exceptions. If it's an easy request and it won't make your life harder, then why not? If someone doesn't want bell peppers in the pasta sauce, then spoon off a little sauce into a separate dish before adding the bell peppers. But if one of your supportive foods is salad, and you live with someone who refuses to eat vegetables, they can fend for themselves from what is in the fridge or freezer.

You should also realize that you don't have to spend a lot of time in the kitchen in order to embrace home cooking and meal planning.

"Between a day job and my kitchen- and health-coaching practice, I work more than full time," Baker relates. "I also do some continuing education, drive carpool, attend sporting events, monitor homework as needed, take kids to appointments, do the shopping and laundry, and carve out time for myself. My husband does the same.

"Yet we manage to put 21 made-from-scratch meals on the table every week - okay, we might eat out once a week," confides Baker. "We generally spend two to four hours on the weekend getting a few things ready for the week, but we make a habit of never cooking for just one meal - that is probably the biggest secret to making more meals from scratch.

"So if you count those weekday hours, you're looking at about seven to ten hours a week to make 21 meals - about half the time most people spend on social media and television," explains Baker. "Want to know another secret? There are a lot of recipes that require almost no hands-on time but a long cooking time: take advantage of those to still be able to take care of your other tasks!"

Cooking doesn't have to be overwhelming, even if you don't have a lot of energy. But if you are going to be successful with taking charge of your wellness, it starts with taking charge of your diet.

If grocery delivery is available in your area, try to take advantage of it. Services like Peapod.com will deliver your groceries right to your door. This can be amazingly useful to POTSies. Using a delivery service means you don't have to go to the store, wander around, lug the groceries, and waste all your energy for the day at the grocery store.

Usually there is an increased cost per item for grocery delivery services, but not having to drive to the store and then waste what energy you do have can make it a good trade off.

Whether you're going to the store or having groceries delivered, make sure you have a stocked pantry so you can always have nutritious, supportive food at the ready. Figure out how many times a week you're going to eat at home. As a POTSie your schedule is probably pretty consistent, but spend some time planning it out just the same.

"Take a look at your schedule for the week and figure out how many dinners you'll be at home. Then work backwards," suggests Dudash. "If you're home 4 nights, you know what you need to plan for. I recommend working in a cook-once-eat-twice recipe and also a slow cooker meal. Make one night of cooking count for at least one lunch and another dinner."

I highly recommend you spend half an hour reviewing your logs and finding your supportive and destructive foods before you being meal planning. This process will be make the actual planning much easier.

Get all your food logs from the first two weeks; the week you were just tracking and the week you started experimenting. Take your pen and strike out every food item that didn't make you feel good. If a food item made you feel sluggish, tired, "blah," unhealthy, etc.-- cross it off. These are destructive foods.

After you have eliminated the foods that are destructive, cross off every typically unhealthy food item that remains. Unhealthy items that might still be on your list include: cake, cookies, pie, ice cream, fries, anything deep fried and greasy like chips or pork rinds.

Now that you have crossed off everything destructive and everything that is typically unhealthy, the foods that are left are the ones that support your health and wellness. These are your core supportive foods, and should be cornerstones of your diet.

It is entirely possible there are no supportive foods on your list.

If that's the case, you may have to make a drastic change in order to only eat food that supports you. This is what I had to do when I went vegetarian. Eating meat was destructive to my health and wellbeing.

Every meal left me feeling disgusted and tired. Giving up meat "cold turkey" wasn't without its challenges as everybody else in my daily life, including my husband, eats meat. The change was quite drastic, but I've never felt better and I haven't looked back.

I'm not saying food that is destructive or typically unhealthy should be avoided at all costs. It's nice to have cake on your birthday, or the occasional bowl of chips. But those foods shouldn't have a large role in your diet.

Now that you have your list of supportive foods, start planning your meals for the coming week. Put the focus on supportive foods. I plan for 3 meals a day with a snack mid-morning and mid-afternoon.

It may be hard to change your eating habits at the drop of a hat, and that's perfectly alright. You can start slowly with your snacks. If you usually have chips for a snack, opt for celery and peanut butter instead. If you usually have fries with your burger, opt for a side salad.

Making sudden, drastic changes in your diet can make it hard for you to stick to long-term, and that is the opposite of what we want. Everything I am teaching is designed to help you make long-term wellness changes. I would rather you make small, incremental changes that last than big, drastic changes that fail after a week.

If you are having trouble adding more supportive foods to your diet, check out the pantry checklist at the end of this chapter. This list is full of foods that are healthy and supportive to us POTSies. But take this list with a grain of salt. If you have noticed something on the list is a destructive food for you – it causes symptoms – then don't eat it. Our bodies are all sensitive and all different. *Listen to yours above all else*.

Remember, your meal planning will be much more effective if you first take the time to discover which foods are supportive and which foods are destructive for you. Remember not to rush your changes. Start slowly, and work your way up. After a few weeks, you will be eating a much healthier and much more supportive diet.

Embracing Breakfast

It can be challenging to make healthy changes in a way that ensures they stick if you do it all at once, so we are going to start slowly.

A lot of people eat the same thing for breakfast every day, and that's largely because in the morning we are on autopilot. Eating the same thing for breakfast every day is one less decision we need to make in the morning when we're groggy.

Modifying your breakfast to a healthier meal might not be very easy, but it's well worth it. Once you get into the routine of eating a healthier breakfast, it's one more health conscious action you will be taking every day, and you won't even realize it.

For a long time, my default breakfast included hardboiled eggs and steel cut oats. Hardboiled eggs are super quick in the morning, but obviously this won't be a good solution if you're vegan (which I am now). If you're not vegan, boil a bunch of eggs on Sunday, and run on autopilot throughout your work week.

Steel cut oats are also super easy in the morning. In a pot the night before, add steel cut oats to filtered water; add a dash of salt and your seasonings. Bring to a boil. Turn down, let simmer for 15 minutes, then turn the heat off and put the lid on. Leave the pan out on the stove overnight. In the morning you will have perfectly cooked steel cut oats. You could also only do it every other day as the oats keep in the fridge for a day or two.

Even if you only eat something light in the morning, eating breakfast can be very helpful. I resisted the idea of eating breakfast for years, but now I love it. Breakfast – even something small and light – gives me a little kick of energy and gets me out of the sleep fog a little bit faster.

Here are a few suggestions:

- Rye muffins with peanut butter
- Green smoothie
- Homemade banana bread
- Protein shake
- Breakfast burritos with tofu
- Scrambled eggs

- Blueberry mousse with chia seeds
- Crisp bread with flaxseed
- Apple peanut butter clusters

You can find these recipes and other resources on my website: 42yogis.com/pots-resources

I recommend mixing it up for the first week until you find a healthy breakfast that suits you. And once you do, try to run on autopilot. When you eat the same thing for breakfast it will be a lot easier for you to get up and get going in the morning. It will be one decision that you won't have to make first thing when you wake up.

Continue logging your food, making sure to write down how you feel after eating your new healthy and easy breakfast. If you've been eating something too sugary in the morning, you may not see a noticeable boost in energy for a few days as it generally takes our bodies a couple days to break the sugar habit.

Changing Up Lunch

For some reason, people don't like to eat the same thing over and over again for lunch every day of the week. Lunch and dinner are times when we can mix it up and explore new foods.

Often, we're working through lunch, or we eat at our desks. I would like to strongly and emphatically discourage this, for one simple reason: when we are eating in front of our work, or while we are doing something else, we stop focusing on the act of eating. *We stop being mindful.*

According to a 2013 study in the *American Journal of Clinical Nutrition* (Robinson E, 2013), people who are distracted during lunch feel full less quickly than people who are mindful. Additionally, they ate more later in the day to make up for not feeling full during lunch.

If you're pressed for time, you can still eat mindfully. Take 10-15 minutes for your lunch, and eat slowly and purposefully. Turn your phone to silent, close your laptop. Pay attention to how the food feels in your mouth. Be aware of the textures and the flavors.

Eat slowly, and notice when you start to get full. It might very well be before you are finished with the meal. That's perfectly fine. If you are trying to reduce calories, stop before you are completely full and drink a full glass of water. Drinking water will fill you up and trick your brain into thinking you ate more than you did, without the tedium of counting calories.

Lunch doesn't have to be a big ordeal if you don't want it to be. Here are some simple and easy to prepare lunch suggestions:

- Fresh veggies and hummus
- Veggie wrap
- Fresh veggies and quinoa
- Artichoke parmesan dip with veggies and pita
- Carrot salad
- Quinoa pear salad
- Quinoa with sweet potatoes and tofu
- Mediterranean tomato couscous
- Wild rice and quinoa

You can find these recipes and other resources on my website: 42yogis.com/pots-resources

I encourage you to plan your lunches ahead of time focusing on meals that are easy to prepare, and that can be prepared in advance.

Modifying Dinner

At this point, you have modified your snacks, breakfast, and lunch with healthier choices. Now, we're going to tackle dinner, but we're also going to adjust your breakfast and lunch a little bit.

Our meals usually look something like this:

We eat a moderately light breakfast, a light lunch, and a big dinner. But this isn't necessarily the best system.

Now I want you to make your breakfast and lunch larger than your dinner. Of course, they should still be healthy meals consisting of foods you identified that didn't cause flares, but you should have more calories than you do for dinner.

The reason is because most of us go to bed within a few hours of dinner. Professor Carl Johnson of Vanderbilt University discovered that when we ingest a lot of calories for dinner and then we don't use them, they usually get stored as fat.

Start getting into the practice of having a larger breakfast and a larger lunch, but smaller dinner. This is difficult, and can take a lot of work. If you're like me and you're not hungry in the morning, you'll have to overcome the feeling of forcing yourself to eat in the morning. If that's the case, start small and work your way up.

Start your evening meal by drinking a full glass of water before you eat. This will help you feel fuller faster, and will hopefully reduce the postprandial hypotension you may be experiencing after dinner.

Try to eat mindfully. Don't sit in front of the TV or your computer (something I'm totally guilty of from time to time), and concentrate on the meal at hand.

As with lunch, eat mindfully. Eat slowly and purposefully. Turn your phone to silent, turn the TV off.

In addition to adjusting the sizes of your meals, also begin to adjust what you're making for dinner. I encourage you to plan your dinners ahead of time focusing on meals that are easy to prepare. If cooking dinner turns out to be an ordeal, you will become more and more likely to opt for something unhealthy.

Continue logging your food, making sure to write down how you feel after eating your new healthy and smaller dinner.

If you're looking for some great cookbooks I recommend these, which are all books I have and use regularly:

The American Diabetes Vegetarian Cookbook by Steven Petusevsky
Simple Recipes for Joy by Sharon Gannon
The Lusty Vegan by Ayinde Howell

Ultimate Pantry Checklist for POTSies

Vegetables	
<ul><li>Artichokes</li><li>Asparagus</li><li>Bean Sprouts</li><li>Beets</li><li>Broccoli</li><li>Cabbage</li><li>Carrots</li><li>Celery</li><li>Corn</li><li>Cucumbers</li><li>Eggplant</li><li>Garlic</li><li>Ginger</li><li>Green Beans</li><li>Jicama</li><li>Kale</li><li>Leeks</li><li>Onions</li><li>Parsnips</li><li>Peas</li><li>Potatoes, white and sweet</li><li>Spinach</li><li>Tomatoes</li><li>Zucchini</li></ul>	Keeping fresh and frozen vegetables in your house is an important part of any healthy diet. If you have fresh veggies around, you'll be more likely to eat them. I recommend favoring fresh veggies wherever possible. Fresh vegetables are full of nutrients that are lost when vegetables are cooked or canned. I like to keep pre-cut fresh vegetables in the house for a quick and healthy snack.

Fruit	
<ul><li>Apples</li><li>Apricots</li><li>Bananas</li><li>Blueberries</li><li>Cherries</li><li>Cranberries</li><li>Grapefruit</li><li>Lemon</li><li>Lime</li><li>Mango</li><li>Melon</li><li>Peaches</li><li>Pears</li><li>Pineapples</li><li>Raisins</li><li>Raspberries</li><li>Strawberries</li></ul>	Fruit not only makes for a good snack and tasty dessert, but it's also a great way to add some variety to a savory dish. I love adding pineapple to yellow curry, dried cranberries to oatmeal, and cherries to rice. The fruits here are chosen because of their diverse uses, and ease of storage. Every fruit on this list can be a snack, ingredient in a desert, added to a savory recipe, blended with other fruits and veggies as a nutritious smoothie, or used in fruit salad.

Dry Goods	
<ul><li>Beans, black</li><li>Beans, garbanzo</li><li>Beans, pinto</li><li>Breadcrumbs, plain or panko</li><li>Chia seeds</li><li>Dried Apricots</li><li>Dried Cherries</li><li>Dried Cranberries</li><li>Flax seed</li><li>Lentils</li><li>Millet</li><li>Noodles, quinoa</li><li>Noodles, ramen</li><li>Noodles, rice</li><li>Oats, steel cut</li><li>Oats, rolled</li><li>Pasta</li><li>Peanuts</li><li>Polenta</li><li>Quinoa</li><li>Rice</li><li>Sunflower Seeds</li></ul>	Keeping a variety of dry goods on hand will make your meal planning easier. Dried fruit can be used in granola, oatmeal, or baking. Chia seeds, flax seed, and sunflower seeds can be added to items like yogurt or peanut butter. I prefer quinoa, ramen, and rice noodles because of the lower gluten content. Traditional pasta is perfectly fine if gluten isn't a concern for you.

Cans and Jars	
<ul><li>Apple Butter</li><li>Applesauce</li><li>Beans, black</li><li>Beans, cannellini</li><li>Beans, garbanzo</li><li>Hominy</li><li>Jams</li><li>Olives</li><li>Peanut Butter</li><li>Pickles</li><li>Roasted Red Peppers</li><li>Tomatoes, San Marzano</li><li>Tomato Sauce</li><li>Vegetable Broth</li></ul>	Canned goods are great because they can be used easily with minimal prep. While I keep dried beans in the house, I also keep canned beans for the times when I forget to soak beans the day before. San Marzano tomatoes are versatile, delicious, plum tomatoes that are canned without the skins. You can chop them as small as you like. San Marzano tomatoes are often regarded to be the best plum tomatoes on the market. Many canned food brands have San Marzano tomatoes.

Sweeteners	
<ul><li>Agave</li><li>Honey</li><li>Maple Syrup</li></ul>**Baking Sweeteners**<ul><li>Granulated sugar</li><li>Brown sugar</li><li>Confectioners' sugar</li></ul>	In regular cooking if something calls for a sweetener, I use one of these three. Often these three sweeteners have more carbs than sugar, but you often need less to achieve the same level of sweetness. Agave is my personal favorite. If you're baking, you often need granulated sugar for a variety of functions, so it is good to have some on hand.

Condiments, Vinegars, Oils, and Spices	
<ul><li>Apple Cider Vinegar</li><li>Balsamic Vinegar</li><li>Balti Seasoning</li><li>Basil</li><li>Cilantro</li><li>Cinnamon</li><li>Chili Powder</li><li>Coconut Oil</li><li>Curry Powder</li><li>Dill</li><li>Ketchup</li><li>Ginger, dried</li><li>Mustard</li><li>Olive Oil</li></ul>	<ul><li>Oregano</li><li>Paprika</li><li>Parsley</li><li>Pepper</li><li>Rosemary</li><li>Sage</li><li>Sambal Oelek</li><li>Sea Salt</li><li>Soy Sauce</li><li>Sriracha</li><li>Tamari</li><li>Tamarind</li><li>Thyme</li></ul>

Meat Substitutes	(If you are eliminating or limiting meat)
<ul><li>Black Bean Burgers</li><li>Soy Bacon</li><li>Soy Beef</li><li>Soy Chicken</li><li>Soy Chorizo</li><li>Soy Sausage</li><li>Tofu</li><li>TVP</li><li>Veggie Burgers</li></ul>	A lot of companies are coming out with meat alternatives. In national grocery stores you can find soy-based alternatives to most meat.

Water

When you have POTS, you may need to drink at least 2-3 liters of water each and every day!

This may sound simple, and it may not sound like much of a challenge, but drinking water can have a huge impact on your health. Some benefits of drinking enough water are:

- It's good for your skin.
- It's good for your digestion, making it easier for you to process food and eliminate waste.
- Water can increase your brain power. Studies show when you have enough water, your reaction time, visual processing, and verbal recognition might all increase.
- Water makes you happier. Studies show people become tense, irritable, stressed out, and even sad when dehydrated. Even a 1.5% decrease in hydration can start to cause these feelings.

There are days when I drink 4 liters of water or more. But I have discovered drinking too much water can be detrimental as well-- I have to use the bathroom all the time which can interrupt my precious sleep.

In general, I aim for 2L-3L per day. In my book, tea counts as water. I don't count coffee because it's dehydrating. Some experts believe one gets slightly more water than they lose when drinking coffee, but the evidence isn't conclusive.

I don't count soda because I consider soda primarily unhealthy for me, and shouldn't be drinking it anyway. Some doctors believe juice counts, although I don't drink juice often because most juice commercially available is mainly sugar, and I don't like sugar. (If I had a juicer and could make low-sugar juices retaining the fruits' fiber, this might be completely different.)

I do sometimes drink Gatorade because of the electrolyte content. Electrolytes help me stay functional, but the sugar in Gatorade is a problem for me.

The Institute of Medicine, a division of the National Academies of Sciences, Engineering, and Medicine, determined that an adequate intake (AI) for men is roughly 3 liters a day. The AI for women is roughly 2.2 liters. I think of it as four - six 16.9 ounce bottles. Each 16.9 ounce bottle is equal to 500 ml. There is nothing wrong with drinking 3L daily. It is not an unhealthy amount over the course of 24 hours.

If you exercise, you should have an additional 400 ml – 600 ml for every 30 minutes of sweat-inducing exercise. Hot weather, humid weather, and higher elevations can all increase the rate at which you lose water. You should drink 500 ml – 1000 ml more water if you live in any of these environments.

Too much water in too short a period of time can be bad for you, and even cause death. When you drink too much water (6L or more) within too short of a window of time (a couple hours), you're depriving your body of necessary electrolytes like salt, potassium, and magnesium. The kidneys control how rapidly electrolytes and other solutes are flushed out of the body, but if you drink too much water in too short an amount of time, the kidneys become overwhelmed.

Consuming too much water too quickly is rare. I know that's definitely not my problem; my problem is not drinking enough water throughout the day.

You can log your water intake on many smartphone apps. I used to use Waterlogged, but now I log it in my FitBit. You can write it down in a notebook or on a Post-It. How you track your water isn't important as long as you know at the end of the day how much water you drank.

I have struggled with drinking enough water for a very long time. I have to consciously work at it to make sure I'm really drinking enough. Over the years I have found 10 tips to make it easier. Here they are:

1. Find your perfect temperature. I like sipping on hot water with ginger throughout the day (in the Ayurveda fashion), which does help keep me drinking water. I also really enjoy drinking room temperature

water. I do not like drinking ice cold water, but a lot of people do. It's a matter of finding what works for you. At what temperature are you most likely to drink water? Find that temperature and make sure to always have a vessel of water at that temperature nearby for you to sip on.

2. Find your perfect vessel. I have multiple drinking vessels for multiple purposes. I have my pretty 42Yogis blue aluminum Sigg bottle which is great for when I'm on the go. My Sigg is lightweight, even when full of water, so it accompanies me to yoga class or the gym. I have a glass Snapware bottle that I use throughout the day for room-temperature water. And I have an insulated glass Cupanion bottle that I use for hot tea (I count herbal tea as water), and hot water with lemon and ginger.

3. There's an app for that. There's an app for everything and anything. But by far the most useful app for me is the one that tracks my water consumption. There are several on the market. If you have a FitBit, you can track your water intake through the FitBit app.

   Or check out Waterlogged because it's a super simple interface. You tell it what your goal is for the day (one day is from 12am-11:59pm), and to log, you simply tap the big glass of water on the screen and enter the ounces. It has quick-set vessels for sizes you use regularly.

4. Start a water support group. Find a support buddy for your water. It could be a colleague, sibling, friend, or spouse. It doesn't matter who it is as long as you're both supportive and committed to hitting your water goal.

5. Drink 16 ounces when you wake up. Keep a glass of water next to your bed and drink it when you first wake up, before you even get out of bed. I learned this awesome little lifehack from entrepreneur Peter Shankman, and it is backed up by Ayurveda and health experts. A glass of water first thing in the morning jump starts your system and gets things moving again after a night of stasis.

6. Drink 16 ounces before a meal. Drinking a big glass of water before a meal has multiple benefits. First, you get another 16 ounces of water. Second, it will make you feel fuller faster, and help prevent you from overeating. There have been studies which indicate drinking water before a meal will speed up your metabolism.

7. Drink 16 ounces of water before a shower. There are multiple theories about whether or not drinking water before a shower is actually helpful in remaining hydrated. Some people even claim drinking a glass of water before a shower will lower blood pressure. I'm hard pressed to find any conclusive studies about this published on the National Institutes of Health. But drinking water before a shower is good if for no other reason, it's yet one more glass of water you get to check off your list.

8. Make water fun. There are people who can drink water all day long and others who get bored and crave variety. If you crave variety, try adding some flavor to your water. I love lemon and ginger. Other tasty water infusions include:

    - Strawberry and mint
    - Strawberry and ginger
    - Raspberries
    - Watermelon
    - Cucumber and mint
    - Cinnamon and ginger
    - Coconut (You can buy coconut water, or if you just want the flavor, stick a piece of coconut meat in your water.)
    - Pineapple
    - Basil and watermelon
    - Cucumber and lime
    - Lemon and lime
    - Lime and cilantro (a personal favorite!)
    - Rose petals
    - Grapefruit and rosemary
    - Kiwi and raspberry
    - Orange and blueberry

9. Refill your vessel as soon as it's empty. Waiting to refill your vessel will mean you don't have water ready to sip on. (See, nothing gets past me!) I find when I don't have water by me, I'm less likely to get out of the chair to go get some when I'm thirsty; especially if I'm in the middle of something, like writing this book, or having a POTS flare.

10. Cleverly placed Post-Its. Posting about your water goal all over the house will remind you to drink water. Added bonus? It may also help your housemates drink more water. I suggest Post-Its in the following locations:

    - On the fridge and/or food pantry: "Are you hungry or thirsty? Drink water before opening me."
    - On your desk: "3L today!" (or whatever your goal is)
    - On the inside of your front door: "Take your water bottle!"

Meditation

Meditation is a great way to find clarity, balance, and sanity in your day. I like to do visual meditations where I visualize my body being filled with health and positive energy as I breathe in. As I exhale, I imagine I am breathing out the pain, discomfort, and anxiety that comes with having POTS.

When I was a kid my parents taught EMT classes to firefighters, and I used to go with them to class. (I loved it, and I think this is where my desire to help people came from.) My parents used to explain to the firefighters about the importance of managing their own stress so they could help patients better. I remember my Mom saying, "Good stress is still stress, and hard on your body." I didn't know what she meant at the time, but I completely get it now.

I am working my butt off trying to make 42Yogis a brand for good and a brand that can change people's lives. I absolutely love my work. I love what I do, and I look forward to working on 42Yogis every single day. But even though I am happy in my work, it is stressful. I consider this "good stress," but my body doesn't differentiate between good stress and bad stress. At the end of the day, it's all stress.

Meditation is an amazing tool for managing stress. It's not magic and it's not a mystery. Meditation activates your parasympathetic nervous system and causes your heart rate to slow, your blood pressure to decrease, and over time meditation starts to change your brain's default mode network.

Your brain's default mode network is a series of regions of your brain that are activated during things like daydreaming, fantasizing, trying to read social cues, remembering facts, and many other things that are required of a waking, but non-attentive, brain. The default mode network is considered your brain's resting state, and it happens when your brain is engaged in these other tasks.

When your brain is active (like when writing a book), your default mode network deactivates.

A study recently published in *Neuroscience and Biobehavioral Reviews* suggests meditation practitioners have structural changes in areas of the default mode network that are not present in non-meditation practitioners. (Kieran C.R. Fox, 2014) Activating the default mode network more regularly is connected to creativity, increased self-perception, and relaxation.

Who doesn't want increased creativity, a better self-image, and to be less stressed?

Start adding meditation to your daily habits of drinking water, changing your language, tracking your food, and simply checking in with your body.

How to Meditate

Meditation practitioners all over the world will tell you that you are capable of achieving peace and serenity. The ability to master meditation will help you find solace in even the most difficult of times.

When you are practicing mindful meditation, you are enabling thoughts to pass through you without aversion or judgment, just acknowledgement and awareness.

There are skills and techniques that you can practice to help you achieve the best mindful mediation session possible. Here are some things you can do to get started.

Step 1: Choosing The Right Place

Choosing the right place is often the most important task for meditation, and also the hardest. You need to find a location where you can focus. Whether it's outside under a tree or in your bedroom, your meditation spot must be quiet, serene, and peaceful. You need to be able to focus your positive energy and let go of the issues that are bogging you down.

You should also consider the environment and atmosphere of the area and decide if it's too dark or too light. I like to meditate outside my house down by the creek, but that's not always the smartest idea, especially during the winter. Any place where you feel comfortable mediating should obviously also have no feeling of danger.

Step 2: Sitting, standing, or walking meditation?

There are so many different ways to meditate, and they all have their value. You can stand, sit, walk, or do variations of these. You must find one position to use and maintain for the duration of your meditation session. Tomorrow you can try something else, and after a week or two of consistent practice you will figure out what method works best for you.

Many practitioners place their hands in their lap or on their thighs. It doesn't matter where you place your hands as long as you can keep them still during your meditation.

Seated
For some of the individuals who are practicing mindfulness meditation, seated has been the most efficient way of calming the mind and relaxing the body. Sitting in a sturdy upright chair with a strong back allows you to focus on the flow of your energy. This is one of the most natural positions for people in the West.

Half Lotus
This is a seated position that many people use as it is much easier to execute than the full lotus. Sit with your buttocks on a cushion or the floor, place one foot on the opposite thigh, and the other foot on the floor beneath the opposite thigh. Be sure that both knees touch the floor and your spine doesn't tilt to one side.

Full Lotus
This is one of the most famous meditation postures and is practiced around the world. With your buttocks on a cushion or the floor, cross your left foot over your right thigh and your right foot over your left thigh. This has also

been considered to be the most stable of all the poses, but it can take some practice to work up to it.

Standing

This upright position focuses on the energy flowing to your whole body. It is important to maintain a solid base and keep your feet planted firmly on the floor, and reach through the ground with your heels.

Standing is one of the most difficult postures as you have to focus on maintaining a strong foundation and keeping balance while mediating.

Walking

Walking meditation can be done alone, or at the end of your seated or standing meditation to get your blood flowing. Walking meditation focuses on your intention to move in a slower pace, allowing you to concentrate on your body, and your mind.

Step 3: Getting Relaxed

You need to decide whether to close your eyes or leave them open. When you close your eyes it can give you the sensation of daydreaming or falling asleep.

When your eyes are widely open you can be easily distracted by external movements, noises, and lights. This can make you lose concentration.

Some meditation practitioners are able to widen their eyes and soften their focus. This allows them to stare off into space and not be distracted by the feeling of falling asleep.

You can place your hands anywhere, just as long as you feel comfortable and your hands will not have any tension that may lead to disrupting you.

When you have decided which posture to use, you can start to meditate by taking a few deep breaths, and letting your body relax with each exhale. After three to five deep inhalations and exhalations return to your normal breathing pattern.

Getting relaxed is the secret to meditation, and once you have accomplished it, you have another challenge: maintaining it. Try focusing on your breath while allowing your thoughts to come, and your thoughts to go. Do not focus on them, only acknowledge that they exist.

The goal of mindfulness meditation should be to observe yourself and understand how the body and mind interact. Maintaining a regular meditation practice will help you release the stress, fear, and anxiety that are keeping you from reaching your true potential.

Meditation Step by Step

Find a selection of guided meditations at 42yogis.com/pots-resources.

1. Find a place where you won't be disturbed for 6 minutes. It doesn't matter where this place is as long as you can sit comfortably, and be left alone.
2. Find your comfortable seat, whether it's on the floor cross-legged, or sitting straight up in a chair. Some people can even meditate lying down, but you run the risk of falling asleep.
3. Silence your phone completely (airplane mode is perfect here), and set a timer for 5 minutes.
4. Close your eyes.
5. Take a deep breath in and then exhale completely.
6. On your next breath, imagine your body is a vessel and air is water. Imagine you are filling your body with air starting at the bottom. Breathe into your abdomen, then your lungs, then your upper chest. Allow your abdomen and chest to expand as you inhale.
7. On your exhale, imagine you are pouring water out the top of a vessel. Empty the air from the top of your chest first, then your abdomen, and then your chest.
8. Continue this breathing exercise at your own pace, moving as slowly as you need to until your timer goes off.
9. When the timer goes off, slowly come back to the room, and return to natural breath. Stretch your arms and legs, and return to the world filled with serenity.

If you find your mind wandering, don't worry. That's normal. It can take years to train your mind not to wander during meditation. Acknowledge your mind is wandering. Acknowledge the thought as it comes into your consciousness, and simply let it go. Let it leave your consciousness, and return your focus to your breath.

To remain focused on your breath and get an extra boost of positive energy try this:

- As you inhale, imagine you are filling your body with light and positivity.

  As you exhale, imagine you are pouring out all the negativity and toxins that have built up in your body.

Meditation for making healthier choices

- Set a timer for 5 minutes, sit in a comfortable position, close your eyes.
- Inhale deeply, exhale completely.
- On your next inhalation, envision the idea of healthy choices. Breathe normally, but focus on this idea for a moment.
- On your next exhalation, envision some unhealthy choices you keep making. Envision without guilt.
- On your next inhalation, breathe in acceptance of your past choices, resolving to move forward.
- On your next exhalation, breathe out all the guilt, remorse or sadness associated with unhealthy choices in the past.
- For the remainder of your meditation, every time you inhale, breathe in acceptance and strengthen your resolve to move forward. Every time you exhale, exhale the negative feelings that have built up as a result of unhealthy choices.

Meditation for Abundant Energy

- Set a timer for 5 minutes, sit in a comfortable position, close your eyes.
- Inhale deeply, exhale completely.
- On your next inhalation, envision what energy means to you.
- On your exhalation, breathe out exhaustion. Breathe out tiredness.
- On your next inhalation, breathe in energizing energy. Not just positive energy, but the kind of energizing energy that makes you want to get up and dance.
- For the remainder of your meditation, every time you inhale, breathe in that energizing energy. Every time you exhale, exhale the tiredness that has built up in your body.

Meditation for Clearing Blocks

- Set a timer for 5 minutes, sit in a comfortable position, close your eyes.
- Inhale deeply, exhale completely.
- On your next inhalation, envision what being healthy means to you. What do you think it will feel like? How will you feel when you achieve your wellness goals?
- On your exhalation, breathe out negativity you have had about your wellness or health. Breathe out the negative energy that has been holding you back and keeping you from achieving your goals.
- On your next inhalation, bring back that positive feeling you want to achieve with wellness. Hold onto that feeling. Feel the light and the warmth of being healthy.
- For the remainder of your meditation, every time you inhale, breathe in that warmth, that light. Strengthen your resolve to conquer your goals in entirety. Every time you exhale, exhale the negativity that has built up in your body from previous roadblocks or setbacks.

Meditation for Looking Back

- Set a timer for 5 minutes, sit in a comfortable position, close your eyes.
- Inhale deeply, exhale completely.
- On your next inhalation remember what you felt like 6 weeks ago. Your energy levels, your focus, your determination.
- On your exhalation, breathe out any negativity associated with that feeling.
- On your next inhalation, think about how you feel today. Notice your energy, ability to focus, how determined you are to be healthy.
- For the remainder of your meditation, focus on how much healthier you feel today than you did at the beginning of this program.

Mantras

Reciting mantras can be very meditative, and you may find this helpful in calming your mind. Below are some of my favorites.

I deserve food that I enjoy, that supports my well-being. This week I will listen to my body and start making meal choices that support my immediate and long term wellness.

I deserve loving kindness. This week I will begin to look at my life, my body, and my mind with love. I will begin to make a plan for the abundant wellness I deserve.

I deserve to feel alive, vibrant, and youthful! I deserve a life of abundant energy, and a body that is healthy enough to keep up with my spirit!

I deserve deeply restorative sleep that supports my wellbeing, and leaves me feeling refreshed, and energized.

I deserve abundant wellness, and I deserve to surround myself with people who support my healthy choices.

Fitness

Important: Before you undertake any new fitness regimen, talk to your trusted medical team.

POTSies tend to lose strength because we have to live modified lives. We can't carry heavy things; we can't work out like most people, so as a result we lose muscle mass.

Muscle mass has a wonderful side-effect of making us feel happier and more confident. When we feel stronger physically we become less discouraged by POTS. Strength training has many benefits, including protecting bone mass and muscle mass, and reducing blood sugar.

The American Diabetes Association recommends those who have type 2 diabetes engage in strength training exercises to increase blood sugar control. "Strength training (also called resistance training) makes your body more sensitive to insulin and can lower blood glucose." (American Diabetes Association, 2015)

Even if you do not have diabetes, this can be helpful to dysautonomia patients as insulin can increase the resting heart rate, as Dr. Bernard Ashby, explained in an earlier chapter.

Another benefit is that strength training has also been shown to reduce abdominal fat in women. (Treuth, 1995) If you've been frustrated that you can't budge stubborn belly fat because of your POTS limitations, strength training can help.

At the time of this writing, I have lost 27 pounds due to my tightly controlled diet, strength training, and yoga. I have done very little jogging in this process. Below are the exercises I do on a regular basis.

Planks

Planks are a powerful way to build strength in your arms and core. Plank is an isometric exercise. The more planks you do, the stronger you'll get. There are several modifications, but the most common is simply the top part of a pushup.

1. Lay on your yoga mat face down.
2. Place your hands under your shoulders and tuck your toes.
3. Press into your hands and lift up until your body is parallel to the floor, arms straight.

An easier modification:
1. Start on your hands and knees with your knees hip width apart and your arms straight.
2. Reach your legs back behind you, tucking your toes.

Regardless of how you get into plank, tighten your abs, and draw your belly button towards your spine to get that core toning. In the beginning it may be hard for you to hold plank for too long, but that's OK. Listen to your body.

Forearm Plank

Want to increase core strength? Bust out forearm plank.

Forearm plank is an intense core strengthener. You come into forearm plank the same way as plank, but instead of balancing on your hands, you come down onto your forearms with your fingers pointing straight ahead.

This is an intense core strengthener, and unless you already have good core strength, you won't be able to hold forearm plank as long as plank, but don't worry about that. Work your way up.

Dumbbell Bicep Curls

Using light free weights, you can increase strength in your arms, which can make annoying tasks like carrying a laundry basket a lot easier.

1. Stand straight with a dumbbell in your hand, arm straight down.

2. Keep your elbows close to your torso (my elbows line up with my waistline, and I use that as my reference point).
3. Keeping your upper arm straight, bend your elbow, and bring the weight up to your shoulder.
4. Release.
5. Repeat 11 times then switch sides.

I do 12 reps of dumbbell bicep curls per set, and I will do between one and three sets based on my exhaustion level and the weight I am using. The weight varies between 5 pounds and 10 pounds.

Variation: Hammer Curl
A hammer curl is very similar to a dumbbell curl, but you bring the weight across your body. Instead of keeping your arm straight and bringing the weight towards your shoulder, bend across your body so the weight touches your opposite collarbone. Repeat for the same number of reps as a dumbbell curl.

Triceps Extensions
Our triceps are often the weakest part of our arms. In the past I laughingly referred to my less-than-firm triceps as Bingo Wings. Doing triceps extensions three times a week has changed that.

You can do triceps extensions sitting down or standing. When you're first starting out with triceps extensions, begin with a dumbbell held in both hands. As you get stronger you can switch to only using one hand.

1. Bring the weight from in front of you to behind your head, still holding with both hands. Elbows pointing up at the ceiling.
2. Slowly straighten your elbows, raising the dumbbell until your elbows, forearms, and upper arms are in a fairly straight line.
3. Lower down.
4. Repeat.

I do 12 reps of triceps extensions per set, and between one and three sets based on my exhaustion level and the weight I am using. The weight varies between 5 pounds and 10 pounds.

Tabata

Tabata is one of the hottest fitness trends right now. Based on High Intensity Interval Training, you can get a good cardiovascular workout and burn calories in just 4 minutes.

Created by Japanese scientist Dr. Izumi Tabata and researchers from the National Institute of Fitness and Sports in Tokyo, the basic Tabata program looks like this:

- Workout as hard as you can for 20 seconds.
- Rest for 30 seconds.
- Repeat until you reach 4 minutes.

As a POTSie, you may want to rest for 60 seconds or even 5 minutes. That's totally fine. The beauty of Tabata is that you can do anything in that 20 second window as long as you are going as hard as you can. You can do jumping jacks, jump rope, run in place, do pushups, kettleball swings, burpees, rows, squats, crunches, you name it.

Tabata has also been shown to increase metabolism. Exercise physiologist Dr. Michele Olson discovered Tabata is far more effective than traditional cardiovascular exercise. During a study Dr. Olson conducted at her lab in at Auburn University of Montgomery, she found it takes 20 minutes of very brisk walking to have the same caloric burn as four minutes of Tabata. (Coats, 2013)

Additionally, Dr. Olson discovered the resting metabolic rate is doubled for up to 30 minutes after a Tabata workout.

I love doing Tabata because I can't do all out cardio for 5-20 minutes most days. I need to do shorter sessions, or bursts, as I've taken to calling it.

Callanetics

My Mom had a Callanetics tape when I was a kid, and I thought it was just fun to do with her. I didn't understand the immense benefits for someone with exercise intolerance until I got older.

Callanetics is a form of low impact exercise based on ballet exercises developed by Callan Pinckney in the 1980s. Instead of high intensity cardio or weight lifting like you see in many forms of exercise, Callanetics involves small, targeted movements to tone the deeper muscles that are often neglected.

By using precise exercises that do not require the exacerbation of the cardiovascular system, you can tone your body in just minutes a day.

I do some Callanetics exercises daily. Because the exercises are not isotonic the muscles do not require a day of rest. I recommend you check out "Callanetics: 10 years younger in 10 hours" on iTunes or Amazon.

Yoga

Despite popular belief, yoga is more than just stretching. Yoga is a mental, physical and spiritual practice that originated in India. Yoga can help increase your flexibility, align your spine, clear your mind, and assist in healthy sleeping patterns. In addition to increasing flexibility and clearing your head, yoga can be very healing.

And America is figuring this out. Yoga has exploded in popularity in the States; it is currently a $27 billion industry.

Chronic discomfort, illness, and pain is known to cause brain anatomy changes and impairments. But according to M. Catherine Bushnell, PhD, scientific director, Division of Intramural Research, National Center for Complementary and Integrative Health at the National Institutes of Health, yoga can helpful for reversing and preventing the negative effects chronic pain can have on your brain. (Weber, 2015)

Bushnell spoke at the American Pain Society's annual meeting and explained there is evidence from studies conducted at NIH/NCCIH that indicate mind-body techniques, such as yoga and meditation, can counteract the effects of pain on the brain's anatomy. "Practicing yoga has the opposite effect on the brain as does chronic pain," said Bushnell. "Some gray matter increases in yogis correspond to duration of yoga practice, which suggests there is a causative link between yoga and gray matter increases."

POTS patients often live in a world clouded by pain and discomfort, and knowing the pain we have to endure on a regular basis can actually alter the anatomy of our brain is a little terrifying.

"Brain anatomy changes may contribute to mood disorders and other affective and cognitive comorbidities of chronic pain. The encouraging news for people with chronic pain is mind-body practices seem to exert a protective effect on brain gray matter that counteracts the neuroanatomical effects of chronic pain," Bushnell added.

"Both POTS and IST can be affected by the increase in catecholamines such as norepinephrine, colloquially referred to as adrenaline," Dr. Bernard Ashby says. "Therefore, yoga may be beneficial in both conditions by counteracting the increased sympathetic activity catecholamine release through increasing parasympathetic activity, the counter balance to sympathetic activity."

Bernard Ashby, M.D. is an attending cardiologist and assistant professor of medicine at Columbia University's Division of Cardiology at Mount Sinai Medical Center. Dr. Ashby earned his medical degree from Cornell University Weill Medical College in New York and studied health policy at Princeton University. He completed his internship and residency at Columbia University Medical Center in New York, where he was also an assistant professor in the department of medicine. He completed his cardiology training at George Washington University Medical Center in Washington, DC, where he was named chief fellow. Dr. Ashby also completed a postdoctoral clinical and research fellowship in vascular medicine at Johns Hopkins University in Baltimore, Maryland.

"Simply put, yoga teaches the body's nervous system to relax," continues Dr. Ashby. "Yoga has been shown to directly decrease catecholamine release and increase parasympathetic activity. In fact, the Vagus nerve, which is responsible for slowing the heart rate, is part of parasympathetic nervous system and can be stimulated with yoga."

Research published in the *European Journal of Preventative Cardiology* has shown yoga can improve cardiovascular health, possibly as much as aerobic exercise.

Yoga has been powerful in helping me get better. Immediately after a yoga practice my cognitive function will be improved, and my stress levels will be lower. I will also be a little bit more flexible.

There are many forms and schools of yoga.

Hatha represents opposing energies. In Sanskrit 'Ha' means sun, and 'tha' means moon. Hatha yoga develops strength - physical and mental - by focusing on the strength building asanas and practices. Traditionally Hatha is a holistic approach to yoga by combining poses (asanas), gestures (mudra), purification processes (shatkriya), breathing (pranayama), and meditation.

Hatha joins slow and gentle movements with deliberate breath work. Often Hatha is recommended for yoga beginners as a way to ease into the yoga lifestyle. Hatha is a good foundation for aspiring yogis as Hatha focuses on perfect alignment.

Anusara is a form of Hatha yoga developed in 1997 in hopes of bringing a more health-oriented yoga to the west. Anusara practice urges practitioners to attain a higher quality of heart and mind. Anusara emphasizes five major alignment principles. When assuming a yoga pose, practitioners make refinements on the pose's alignment by performing the principles in order, and within each principle, there are further refinements.

Judgment is a non-starter in an Anusara class as students of all levels of ability are honored, accepted, and respected for their unique talents. In

Anusara, your actions and movements are often coordinated with your breath. This class is also recommended for beginners.

Also a form of Hatha yoga, <u>Iyengar</u> was developed in the 1970s and focuses on precision and alignment. Iyengar often - but not always - utilizes props like belts and blocks to help practitioners achieve better alignment. Props make the poses accessible to people who have health ailments or are new to yoga while minimizing the risk of injury to all who use them.

Iyengar yoga places emphasis on the sequence in which the poses are practiced. Following this sequence is important to achieve the desired results.

This style of yoga is a good starting point for beginners.

If you are looking for a strong physical practice, consider practicing <u>Ashtanga</u> yoga. Ashtanga is geared towards people who are looking for something a little more rigorous than Hatha. Ashtanga focuses on aligning the breath with the movement with each pose lasting approximately one inhalation or exhalation.

Unlike most yoga forms in the west, Ashtanga Vinyasa asanas are done in a predetermined order. A practice consists of four main sequences that have remained unchanged for decades.

Derived from the traditional form of Ashtanga Vinyasa is <u>Vinyasa Flow</u>, often just called vinyasa. Vinyasa denotes a flowing form of yoga.

In both Ashtanga Vinyasa and Vinyasa Flow, attention is placed on the movement between asanas instead of just perfect alignment.

In the 1970s Bikram Choudhury took the traditional practice of hatha yoga, modified it, and repackaged it as a new fitness franchise. All <u>Bikram</u> classes are the same, and the practitioners perform the same combination of 26 postures and two breathing exercises within 90 minutes every single time.

The poses can't just be performed in your living room though. Bikram must be performed in a 105-degree room with 40% humidity to allow the body to stretch, detoxify, relieve stress, tone, and heal chronic pain.

All Bikram classes are licensed and taught by certified Bikram instructors, and these instructors are required to recite the Bikram dialogue to the class as opposed to demonstrating poses.

Generally, if you're trying to heal, practicing a gentler yoga form like Hatha, two to three times a week can prove beneficial, although I suggest doing yoga – even if just one or two poses – every single day to get into the habit. If you feel like yoga is helping, incorporating four or five longer sessions per week may be better for you. But I do suggest that you try to avoid the more intense forms of yoga, like Bikram or Ashtanga.

After I was doing yoga for a few months I noticed an increase in my lung capacity, relief from back and neck pain, an improved sense of balance, and increased strength. Yoga has so much to offer, but, for POTSies it's not easy to get started.

The first thing you need to be aware of (but you probably already know) is that everything takes longer for us POTSies. That is true of yoga. You have to go at your own pace and listen to your body. What might take a "normal" person one month can take us three.

Don't push it, and don't rush it, or you'll have a flare up. When you're at the edge of your comfort zone, STOP.

Don't push yourself to the point of injury because you think this is how it's "supposed to be."

As a POTSie you can feel injuries more severely the next day, and the pain can trigger a flare up.

Go at your own pace; listen to your body, and most importantly – be consistent. It's far more important you show up to the mat every day than whether or not you quickly master each pose. Consistency builds the habit.

To start, you should set aside an afternoon when you don't have anything planned for the evening. Until you've done yoga a few times and started to feel your body differently, you won't know for sure if you'll have a flare or not. My first two times I had flares, but then I realized I was pushing myself too hard. It's important to remember that yoga is a practice, not a perfection. Go at your own pace, and you will find what works for you. If you're new to yoga, I'd suggest you start sitting on your mat. Until you are used to the movements while also breathing in a controlled manner, standing poses could be dangerous, and flows could be horrendous - especially if you are prone to syncope.

After you get comfortable with seated poses and poses where you have a good, strong base under you, then you can move into standing poses.

Supplies for Getting Started with Yoga

If you don't have a yoga mat, you should get one. It doesn't have to be an expensive one, but it's helpful not to have to rely on carpeting. Carpeting is no fun on the knees, let me tell you! Also, carpeting can cause dangerous slipping.

Your yoga mat will become your best friend. Your yoga mat will support you. Your yoga mat will help you without judgment or concern. Your yoga mat will be there for you.

Make sure the mat you get isn't poorly made or too slippery. I found the mainstream yoga mats that are so common on the market were both too thin and too slippery for me.

I use the Manduka eKO Mat. It is made of all natural rubber, and is not slippery at all. It doesn't slide around on the carpet, and I don't slide around on it when I'm doing yoga. (Get 10% off a Manduka mat with the code 42YOGIS at Manduka.com)

There's a lot to consider when picking out your perfect yoga mat.

Yoga mats that properly support your body and practice are essential to grow in your yoga practice. Yoga mats prevent and decrease injuries that can be caused by slippery surfaces. Yoga mats are used to help create a barrier between the yogi and the floor.

Many students will let you borrow a mat to use during your classes, but I don't recommend going this route. You don't know for sure how clean a mat is until you clean it yourself. To keep your mat clean, there are many yoga mat cleaning supplies on the market, but you can always make your own. (I make my own out of apple cider vinegar, witch hazel, lavender, and tea tree oil.)

To be considered a great yoga mat, it needs to be safe, durable, and comfortable. In my book, to be a perfect yoga mat it should also be environmentally friendly.

The right yoga mat will help you improve your balance and coordination and give you better stability and traction. I didn't believe this until I switched from my flimsy Gaiam to my cushy Manduka. Yoga on the Manduka feels like yoga should feel: safe and secure.

If you care about the planet, selecting an eco yoga mat is a perfect choice as you down dog your way to enlightenment. There are some new brands just getting their eco mats off the ground, but here are three brands that you can't really go wrong with:

- Manduka Eko
- Hugger Mugger
- Jade Yoga Mats

One of the problems with eco-mats is that the materials used are meant to biodegrade. With extensive use, your mat might start to wear out. Manduka mats have a great reputation of not wearing out even after years of use. The Manduka Eko I use is a natural rubber mat, and it has a rather strong scent when you first open it up. You might want to let it air out.

PVC based yoga mats last forever, and literally take years to biodegrade. You get a lot more variety in color when you purchase a mat that's a traditional PVC mat as opposed to an eco-friendly mat. Gaiam offers a wide variety of colors and designs. You should be able to find a mat that suits your personality.

Traditional yoga mats can be purchased for as little as $20, and you can even get one at Walmart or K-Mart. This might be the best route to go if you're a yoga newbie and you're unsure you want to stick with the practice.

When I started yoga I purchased a cheap mat from Walmart because I didn't know if I would like yoga. It was only after a steady and consistent practice (that wasn't being properly supported by the cheap mat) that I upgraded to my Manduka.

If something more natural is up your alley, you can get a yoga mat made out of cotton. A 100% cotton yoga mat may be best if you have allergic reactions to other materials. 100% cotton yoga mats are actually called yoga rugs, and they do have a bit of slippage that can be dangerous. Yoga rugs are best for those who do a slow restorative yoga (like us POTSies), or yin yoga, instead of a lot of flows. As a POTSie I expect you won't be doing very many yoga flows, and that's perfectly fine.

In addition to a mat, you should consider getting a block. Blocks are part of a group of yoga products called props. Blocks are very useful for beginner (and sometimes even advanced) yogis. Blocks give you a lot of support in some poses that might not be quite accessible otherwise. They can be found separately, or in yoga essential kits. I prefer cork blocks personally, but the foam ones are cheaper and work just as well.

Yoga straps are also helpful in making poses more accessible. Straps are often found in beginner's yoga class, and using a strap can make sure you're opening up the joints and muscles enough to benefit from everything that the yoga class has to offer. Straps can be found both in a kit or stand alone.

My Morning Yoga Sequence

- Sun Salutations x 1
- Triangle Pose
- Warrior 1
- Warrior 2
- Reverse Warrior
- Standing Forward Fold

Repeat on the other side, making sure to stretch both legs and both arms equally.

Check out my Yoga for POTSies video at 42yogis.com/pots-resources

My Exercise Plan

I try to exercise every single day at five different parts of my day. Because of my dysautonomia I struggle to do a lot of exercise all at once – even now – and I have found breaking my exercises up into chunks throughout the day makes it much more manageable.

Please keep in mind I have worked my way up to this. I haven't always been able to exercise with this frequency. For a very long time even just a few minutes of exercise would knock me on my butt for the rest of the day. It has taken time to build up to where I am now. I have been conditioning my body and conditioning my nervous system.

Do not expect that you will be able to jump into this right away, and discuss any changes to your exercise with your trusted physician beforehand.

	Sunday	Monday	Tuesday	Wednesday
Morning	Yoga 1-5 min.	Yoga 1-5 min.	Yoga 1-5 min.	Yoga 1-5 min.
Before Lunch	---	Plank, Forearm Plank *1-2 min*	Plank, Forearm Plank *1-2 min*	Plank, Forearm Plank *1-2 min*
Mid-Afternoon	Tabata 4 min.	Tabata 4 min.	Tabata 4 min.	Tabata 4 min.
Evening	---	Hammer Curls, Triceps Extensions *1-3 sets of 12 reps each**	Plank *(as long as I can hold it),* Oblique Crunches *(1-3 sets of 12 on each side)*	Hammer Curls, Triceps Extensions *1-3 sets of 12 reps each**
Before Bed	Callanetics or Barre	Callanetics or Barre	Callanetics or Barre	Callanetics or Barre

	Thursday	Friday	Saturday
Morning	Yoga 1-5 min.	Yoga 1-5 min.	Yoga 1-5 min.
Before Lunch	Plank, Forearm Plank *1-2 min*	Plank, Forearm Plank *1-2 min*	---
Mid- Afternoon	Tabata 4 min.	Tabata 4 min.	Roller Skating, *120 min*
Evening	Plank *(as long as I can hold it)*, Oblique Crunches *(1-3 sets of 12 on each side)*	Hammer Curls, Triceps Extensions *1-3 sets of 12 reps each**	Plank *(as long as I can hold it)*, Oblique Crunches *(1-3 sets of 12 on each side)*
Before Bed	Callanetics or Barre	Callanetics or Barre	Callanetics or Barre

* How many sets I do depends on my energy level at this point. Sometimes I only do one set, sometimes three. The weight I use varies between 5-10 lbs, also depending on my energy level and fatigue.

Modifying My Exercise Plan

Instead of jumping in headfirst, start slowly.

I recommend you work your way up adding in more and more exercise as the months go by. One option is to start with 1-5 minutes of yoga daily and do this for six weeks. Or, if that's too much (or too intimidating), try to do yoga only once per week, and slowly add one more day every week so after seven weeks you are doing seven 1-5 minute yoga sessions per week.

If you are feeling up to it after six weeks, start to add in Callanetics. Do both yoga and a few minutes of Callenetics daily for the next six weeks, and reevaluate.

Only add in more exercise after you have adapted to what you have been doing for several weeks. This may be more than six weeks for you. This may be less than six weeks. Make sure you listen to your body and <u>discuss any changes with your trusted medical professionals beforehand</u>.

Pranayama (Breathing) Exercises

If the idea of doing any yoga or exercise is a little scary for you at this point, you might want to start with pranayama exercises, and work your way up to seated poses. Pranayama exercises – breath control exercises – have been very beneficial to me. Let me explain.

When you get stressed your body is flooded with hormones like cortisol and norepinephrine, which heighten the senses, increase heart rate and blood pressure, and focus your brain's activity. For POTSies this can be detrimental.

Luckily, humans are an enlightened bunch and are learning that stress is something that can be mitigated, even when it cannot be entirely avoided. To help bring a sense of calm to your breathing, you can practice breath control exercises such as Alternate Nostril Breathing and Three Part Breath (Dirgha Pranayama).

A 2012 study concluded, "Long-term alternate nostril breathing (ANB) has been shown to enhance autonomic control of the heart by increasing parasympathetic modulation." (Shreya Ghiya, 2012)

Another study conducted in 2013 said, "...the parasympathetic tone was enhanced appreciably in the participants. The observations of this study suggest that the yogic exercise of A.N.B. influences the parasympathetic nervous system significantly." (Sinha AN, 2013)

When you start exploring pranayama exercises as a POTSie, you may feel light headed or dizzy. This is normal, and it is nothing to be alarmed by. But, this is why it's important to do your pranayama when you're seated on your mat and are not at risk of injury. It has taken me a long time to do pranayama exercises. The secret is to start slowly.

Thanks to pranayama, I can calm myself down mentally. I can refocus my mind if my mind is wandering, and I can slow my heart rate.

Alternate nostril breathing can be particularly effective for POTSies.

Alternate Nostril Breathing Step-By-Step

1. Find a comfortable seat with your back straight and shoulders relaxed.
2. Fold your index finger and middle finger on the right hand, and bring your hand to your face.
3. Place the ring finger alongside the left nostril and the thumb alongside the right nostril.
4. Take a deep breath in, and on your exhalation, gently press your left nostril closed with your ring finger and exhale through the right nostril.
5. Inhale through your right nostril, and as you finish your inhalation, press your right nostril closed, and release your ring finger from the left. Exhale through your left nostril.
6. Keeping your right nostril closed, inhale through the left. As you finish your inhalation, press your left nostril closed, and open the right. Exhale through the right nostril.

This is one round of Alternate Nostril Breathing. Continue in this fashion for another 11 rounds. Remember to inhale through the same nostril you just exhaled through.

Keep your breaths long and slow. Don't force, and don't rush.

Three Part Breath (Dirgha Pranayama)

Dirgha Pranayama is a very soothing exercise that can be done anytime you are feeling stressed or anxious, and can slow down your heart rate. You can even do it in traffic.

1. Start by sitting straight up, shoulders down on your back. Root down into your hips, and try to reach up through the crown of your head.
2. Take a long, deep breath, and let it out.

3. On your next inhalation, draw your breath deep into your belly. It may help to place your hand on your navel. Exhale. Repeat for 2 more breaths.
4. Move your hand up to your lower ribs. As you inhale notice the expansion of your ribs. Exhale. Repeat for 2 more breaths.
5. Move your hand up to your sternum. As you inhale notice the expansion of your chest. Exhale. Repeat for 2 more breaths.

As you do dirgha pranayama more and more you may notice it flows naturally and you no longer need your hand to guide you.

It may be beneficial to envision your body as a vessel and the air as water. Just as you fill the bottom of the vessel when you pour in water, try to do so with your breath.

If you cannot yet control your breath in this manner, don't worry. Often it is a visualization exercise to start, but over time, you'll build up awareness and control of the muscles.

POTS and Travel

I'm writing this chapter in the air over Lake Erie. I'm on a flight from Buffalo to Chicago, and this seems like the perfect time to write about what it's like to be a POTSie who travels regularly.

Making the decision to travel – or not travel – is very much part of lifestyle design, and ultimately the decision comes down to what kind of life you want to live. I, for one, do not want to stay in my small town and never see the world. I can't live like that, and I don't think I should have to just because I have a health problem that makes traveling difficult.

Over the years I have traveled a lot. I usually fly two to five times per year, and I take at least three long road trips per year. There was one year I traveled over 20,000 miles; 10,000 of it by car.

I have long wondered if my inclination toward travel has anything to do with my Romanian gypsy heritage. But the urge - need - to travel is matched by a strong desire to stay home where I'm safe and I can manage my POTS with ease.

So, I clearly have a love/hate relationship with traveling. I love going places, seeing new things, and meeting new people, but I hate the act of traveling. Traveling - whether by air or car - does some unpleasant things to my body, and can cause a POTS flare.

Several years ago I was flying from Upstate NY to California. The airplane sat on the runway in Rochester for several hours, and we had no food or drink. We got to the Newark airport with just a few moments to spare before the last plane to SFO. As if that wasn't bad enough, we had to disembark on the tarmac, and go through security again. I was carrying my laptop and a guitar. I ended up collapsing in a POTS flare in front of a gate counter.

A doctor was nearby and saw what was happening to me, and called 911. I explained it's actually fairly normal for me to have a POTS flare after eight hours without anything to eat or drink, on top of carrying two heavy bags all through the airport!

The Port Authority medics showed up, and said I just had a panic attack. (How many times have you heard *that* as a POTSie?) The airline said I could sleep in the airport until the next flight at 6 am. Luckily, I have some friends in New Jersey, and one of them picked me up and I stayed at his house for the night so I could sleep in an actual bed.

This incident kept me from flying for a few years. But I still needed to travel. So I did what any young woman with a new car would do: I drove across the country.

In the years following the airport incident, I drove 20,000 miles around the country by myself.

What I love about driving is that I have control. I may not have control over the other drivers on the road, and I may not have control over the weather conditions, but if I am starting to feel a flare coming on, I can pull into a rest area or truck stop and take care of it. This is not an option when I'm flying.

There are a number of symptoms that are exacerbated as I travel.

If I am traveling by car:
- General hip discomfort
- Blood pooling in my ankles
- Back pain
- Nausea - especially if driving at night
- Migraines

If I am traveling by air:
- General hip discomfort
- Lower back discomfort
- Blood pooling in my ankles
- Dizziness
- Nausea
- Palpitations
- Headaches

And randomly throughout the flight, my heart rate goes up, my blood pressure drops, my ears need to pop, I get dizzy, and incredibly nauseous. I could never be a pilot.

But are these symptoms enough to keep me from flying? No, because I've learned how to manage them.

Here are my tips for making the most of traveling.

Do some yoga
Getting up and moving before and after a flight can go a long way to maintaining balance while you're traveling. When I am traveling by car, I try to stop every couple hours and do some yoga. Whenever I get out of the car, I do some stretching. This keeps my blood flowing, and can help reduce the pooling in my legs. Yoga also keeps my lower back from feeling compressed and tight.

Do breathing exercises
Whether flying or driving, pranayama exercises (breathing exercises) can go a long way to helping you feel calmer, happier, and less stressed. Pranayama can also help calm your heart rate and bring you back down to a better rate.

Meditate
On a recent flight we went through some pretty horrid turbulence as we were flying through a storm, and I started to freak out a little bit. Meditation helped me keep my calm. When I start to get worried or anxious, I go into a POTS episode. Meditation helps me prevent the anxiety before it starts.

Drink lots of water
This is a tricky since I don't like having to pee on the airplane, but if I let myself get too dehydrated, it's bad news. Just because I don't want to use the tiny, creepy airplane bathroom doesn't mean my body needs any less water. I strive to drink 2L-3L per day minimum, and I still have to maintain this when I travel.

Three hours before travel – whether by car or plane – I try to drink a full liter of water. Crazy? Well, yes, it can be, but this ensures that I have at least 30% of my daily water intake and have had plenty of time to pee before I get stuck in a car or on a plane. In the three hours leading up to travel, I continue to drink water, but very small sips. I find it helps to have sodium in the water to keep my blood volume up.

While I'm driving I continue to drink water, as I can stop at rest areas or truck stops. This is not very efficient, and I have estimated I end up lengthening my road trips by 45-60 minutes, but it keeps me from feeling unwell, so the increase in travel time is worth it.

When I am flying I stop drinking water about 30 minutes before the plane boards. For several minutes – sometimes as many as 30 minutes – you can't get up once the plane is in the air, no matter how much you need to pee. I sip on a bottle of water very slowly throughout the flight. As soon as the pilot announces we are beginning our descent towards the airport, I finish the bottle of water.

If I don't have a connection, after we land I fill my bottle of water again and chug it before even leaving the airport. This goes a long way to ensuring I maintain hydration all throughout the trip.

If I have a connection, I will drink water up until 30 minutes before boarding.

Have connections when possible
Having connections means that while you may very well be traveling for a longer period of time total, each individual flight is probably going to be shorter, and this is useful for POTSies. Having a chance to get off the plane after a couple hours, walk around, chug some water, and eat something often makes the difference between a pleasant experience and a horrifying one.

Personal Development

When you have dysautonomia it can be really hard to feel like a human. Because we are always struggling to feel well, to feel even somewhat functional, we often feel weaker and less than everybody else. It's because of this I am a strong advocate of personal development.

We may have physical challenges to overcome, but we still have so much to offer the world by being ourselves. By embarking on a journey of personal development we can continue to grow our minds and have even more to offer the world.

Personal development is a broad topic that spans a variety of areas including:

- Self-esteem
- Knowledge
- Skills
- Spirituality
- Fitness
- Quality of life

As POTSies I think we should develop ourselves in each of these six areas. Of course, there are more areas where one can develop, but these are the six that I have found are key to remaining balanced and sane as a POTSie.

I use mind mapping to do many things, including visualizing my personal development plan. Here's a small portion of my Personal Development Mind Map.

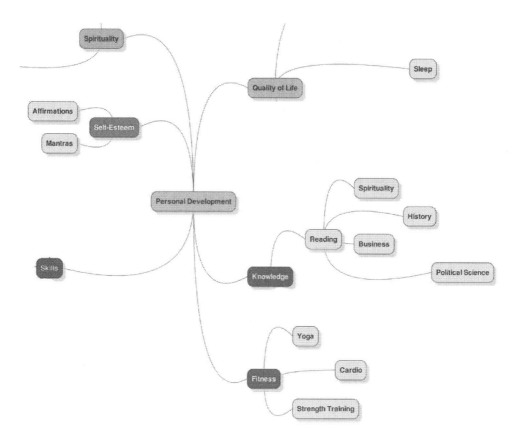

Developing our self-esteem is especially important, as without self-esteem it is very easy to slip into a dark abyss and feel like even less of a person. I'm speaking from personal experience.

Sleep

My sleep has been messed up for years. When I was a kid I used to sleep walk, and it would get me into some dangerous situations. I started sleeping at weird hours; refusing to get on a normal schedule. I felt good at night. I felt awake. The world was quiet, and there was room for me to think, to breathe.

This was only reinforced when I started working as the night editor of a newspaper. I would work from 10 pm - 6 am. I loved it. For years I struggled with breaking this habit. I knew getting on a regular schedule – and a daytime schedule – could be beneficial to my health, but I never quite pushed it to the point of making it happen.

One day, years later, I decided to get up early and see what would happen. I was tired, but, wow, did I feel good! I was in a good mood. I was able to focus at work. I was more present in my daily life. It was fabulous.

I started shifting my schedule so I could get up earlier, and something surprising started to happen: when I started getting up early, my health started improving.

I now naturally awake around 5:45 a.m., and I feel really good when I do. Now when I sleep in I am more likely to have flares.

Now, that being said, your circadian rhythm is not mine. Your body may not do well on a day schedule. Your body may prefer the night. And that's perfectly fine. But here's something we all need: a regular sleep schedule.

Having a regular sleep schedule is important to POTSies – imperative, I would argue. Everything else falls into place when we have a sleep schedule. It is easier to manage our day. Once a sleep schedule has been put in place, we can have a meal schedule. Both a sleep schedule and a meal schedule are important to keep our hormones in balance. Our sleep plays a big role in our wellness; bigger than you might think.

According to a 2006 study, not getting enough sleep can alter our insulin resistance, which is associated with an increased risk of developing type 2 diabetes. (Knutson, 2006)

Sleep deprivation is also linked to a greater risk of catching a cold as indicated by a 2009 study. (Sheldon Cohen, 2009) When I get a cold, I spend the entire time I am sick in a POTS flare. In addition to being congested, and running a fever, I spend a significant amount of time with palpitations and dizziness.

Beyond the physical health benefits of getting enough sleep, it has also been found that getting enough sleep will improve our mood. Insufficient sleep can cause depression, anxiety, and irritability. (Dinges DF, 1997)

When we aren't getting enough sleep our health suffers and our mood suffers. A bad mood makes us less likely to do what is necessary to take care of ourselves, which makes our health suffer even further. When our health suffers, our mood gets worse. It's a vicious cycle.

But it is a cycle that you can break.

For me it all started with my pillow. I got a memory foam pillow three years ago that supports my neck. It's been three years and the pillow is still amazing. Making that one simple change keeps me from waking up with a stiff neck and from tossing and turning at night.

Dr. Robert S. Rosenberg, Board Certified Sleep Medicine Physician and author of *Sleep Soundly Every Night, Feel Fantastic Every Day,* knows what it takes to get better sleep and shared some tips with me. One of the issues is something we are all familiar with, and that is blue light. Computers, mobile phones, iPads, tablets, and TV all emit blue light that can disturb your sleep.

"Blue light is the most disturbing light when trying to go to sleep because it immediately shuts down your production of melatonin, the major sleep hormone that we produce at night," says Dr. Rosenberg.

Limit your blue light exposure for 2 hours before bedtime.

Another common disturbance of sleep is caffeine. For those of us who are chronically fatigued caffeine can be a huge help in making sure we are functional throughout the day.

Limiting caffeine may be something you're already doing as a POTSie, as it can increase our heart rate, or you could be drinking caffeine to combat the fatigue you feel during the day, but if you are having difficulty with sleep, you should take a look at how much caffeine you are drinking.

"Many of us fail to realize how much caffeine can impair our ability to get to sleep and remain asleep," Dr. Rosenberg explains. "Most of us take four to six hours to metabolize caffeine. However, many of us may take much longer. Caffeine blocks the ability of a sleep-promoting chemical called adenosine to work."

Exercise is also very helpful. Studies indicate those who exercise throughout the day sleep better than those who do not. (Pasanen TP, 2013) As a POTsie this may be challenging for you, but I have found even just a little bit of exercise (even just two minutes of exercise) can help me sleep better. You could sit on the edge of your bed and do a few leg lifts, a few stretches, and still sleep a little bit better.

By incorporating these ideas, I've been able to attain better sleep. Try some of them and you might be surprised!

A Final Word of Encouragement

Yes, the road to where I am today has been long and difficult. As you've seen, many, many things have gone into this totally new way of life. But it is a life largely free of POTS symptoms.

When I look back on that girl who could barely go up a flight of stairs, I am amazed at how far I've come. I never thought I'd be able to honestly say: I love my life!

It is my hope that you, too, can create a framework for yourself that empowers and supports who you are and who you can become; a framework that helps you manage your life with POTS.

Resources

Go to 42yogis.com/pots-resources to get a list of resources that can be helpful on your journey. This includes my POTS yoga video, cookbook recommendations, mantras, meditations, and more.

References

American Diabetes Association. (2015, May 19). *What We Recommend.* Retrieved from American Diabetes Association: http://www.diabetes.org/food-and-fitness/fitness/types-of-activity/what-we-recommend.html

Chu, P. (2014, December 15). *The effectiveness of yoga in modifying risk factors for cardiovascular disease and metabolic syndrome: A systematic review and meta-analysis of randomized controlled trials.* Retrieved from Sage Pub: http://cpr.sagepub.com/content/early/2014/12/02/2047487314562741

Coats, J. (2013, June 14). *AUM's Michele Olson finds four-minute workout more effective than traditional cardio, doubles metabolic rate.* Retrieved from AUM: http://www.aum.edu/news-events/2013/06/14/aum-s-michele-olson-finds-four-minute-workout-more-effective-than-traditional-cardio-doubles-metabolic-rate

Dinges DF, e. a. (1997, April 20). *Cumulative sleepiness, mood disturbance, and psychomotor vigilance performance decrements during a week of sleep restricted to 4-5 hours per night.* Retrieved from National Institutes of Health: http://www.ncbi.nlm.nih.gov/pubmed/9231952

Grubb, B. P. (2002). The Postural Tachycardia Syndrome: A Brief Review of Etiology, Diagnosis and Treatment.

Howraa Abed, P. A.-X. (2012). *Diagnosis and management of postural orthostatic tachycardia syndrome: A brief review*. Retrieved from National Institutes of Health: http://www.ncbi.nlm.nih.gov/pmc/articles/PMC3390096/

Kieran C.R. Fox, S. N. (2014, June). *Is meditation associated with altered brain structure? A systematic review and meta-analysis of morphometric neuroimaging in meditation practitioners*. Retrieved from Science Direct: http://www.sciencedirect.com/science/article/pii/S01497634140007 24

Knutson, K. L. (2006, September 18). *Role of Sleep Duration and Quality in the Risk and Severity of Type 2 Diabetes Mellitus*. Retrieved from JAMA Internal Medicine: http://archinte.jamanetwork.com/article.aspx?articleid=410883

Levesque, William R., J.S. (2015, March 7). *2014 Osceola Fundamental High valedictorian home from MIT found dead at TIA*. Retrieved from Tampa Bay Times: http://www.tampabay.com/news/publicsafety/2014-osceola-high-school-valedictorian-dies-while-home-from-mit/2220461

Maltz, M. (2001). *The New Psycho-Cybernetics*. New York: Penguin Putnam.

Pasanen TP, T. L. (2013, November 6). *The relationship between perceived health and physical activity indoors, outdoors in built environments, and outdoors in nature*. Retrieved from NIH: http://www.ncbi.nlm.nih.gov/pubmed/25044598

Robinson E, A. P. (2013, April). *Eating attentively: a systematic review and meta-analysis of the effect of food intake memory and awareness on eating*. Retrieved from National Institutes of Health: http://www.ncbi.nlm.nih.gov/pubmed/23446890

Sheldon Cohen, e. a. (2009, January 12). *Sleep Habits and Susceptibility to the Common Cold*. Retrieved from JAMA Internal Medicine: http://archinte.jamanetwork.com/article.aspx?articleid=414701&res ultClick=24

Shreya Ghiya, C. M. (2012, January). *Influence of alternate nostril breathing on heart rate variability in non-practitioners of yogic breathing*. Retrieved from NIH: http://www.ncbi.nlm.nih.gov/pmc/articles/PMC3276936/

Sinha N, D. D. (2013, May 7). *Assessment of the effects of pranayama/alternate nostril breathing on the parasympathetic nervous system in young adults.* Retrieved from NIH: http://www.ncbi.nlm.nih.gov/pubmed/23814719

Soliman, Kamal et. al. *Postural orthostatic tachycardia syndrome (POTS): a diagnostic dilemma.* Retrieved from British Journal of Cardiology: http://bjcardio.co.uk/2010/02/postural-orthostatic-tachycardia-syndrome-pots-a-diagnostic-dilemma/

Treuth, M. (1995, April 1). *Reduction in intra-abdominal adipose tissue after strength training in older women.* Retrieved from Journal of Applied Physiology: http://jap.physiology.org/content/78/4/1425

Understanding the Stress Response. (2011, March 1). Retrieved from Harvard: http://www.health.harvard.edu/staying-healthy/understanding-the-stress-response

Weber, C. (2015, May 15). *Yoga and Chronic Pain Have Opposite Effects on Brain Gray Matter.* Retrieved from American Pain Society: http://americanpainsociety.org/about-us/press-room/yoga-bushnell

What I Dysautonomia. (2012). Retrieved from Dysautonomia International: http://www.dysautonomiainternational.org/page.php?ID=34

About the Author

Ysmay Walsh is a yoga teacher, business coach and artist, who attempts to prevail over dysautonomia every day. She makes her home in Upstate New York.

Contact Ysmay

Email: ysmay@42yogis.com

Website: 42yogis.com

Made in the USA
Coppell, TX
20 February 2022

73838767R00057